Computational Immunology: Models and Tools

Computational Immunology: Models and Tools

Edited by
Josep Bassaganya-Riera
Nutritional Immunology and Molecular Medicine Laboratory,
Virginia Bioinformatics Institute, Virginia Tech,
Blacksburg, VA, USA

AMSTERDAM • BOSTON • HEIDELBERG • LONDON
NEW YORK • OXFORD • PARIS • SAN DIEGO
SAN FRANCISCO • SINGAPORE • SYDNEY • TOKYO

Academic Press is an imprint of Elsevier

Academic Press is an imprint of Elsevier
125, London Wall, EC2Y 5AS.
525 B Street, Suite 1800, San Diego, CA 92101-4495, USA
225 Wyman Street, Waltham, MA 02451, USA
The Boulevard, Langford Lane, Kidlington, Oxford OX5 1GB, UK

Notices
Knowledge and best practice in this field are constantly changing. As new research and experience broaden our understanding, changes in research methods or professional practices, may become necessary.

Practitioners and researchers must always rely on their own experience and knowledge in evaluating and using any information or methods described herein. In using such information or methods they should be mindful of their own safety and the safety of others, including parties for whom they have a professional responsibility.

To the fullest extent of the law, neither the Publisher nor the authors, contributors, or editors, assume any liability for any injury and/or damage to persons or property as a matter of products liability, negligence or otherwise, or from any use or operation of any methods, products, instructions, or ideas contained in the material herein.

ISBN: 978-0-12-803697-6

Library of Congress Cataloging-in-Publication Data
A catalog record for this book is available from the Library of Congress

British Library Cataloguing-in-Publication Data
A catalogue record for this book is available from the British Library

For Information on all Academic Press publications
visit our website at http://store.elsevier.com/

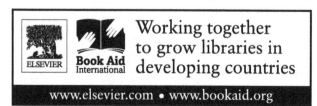

Working together
to grow libraries in
developing countries

www.elsevier.com • www.bookaid.org

Cover Designer: MIEP Team

CONTENTS

Chapter 4 Immunoinformatics Cyberinfrastructure for Modeling and Analytics **45**

*Stefan Hoops, Bruno W. Sobral, Pawel Michalak, Vida Abedi,
Barbara Kronsteiner, Raquel Hontecillas, Monica Viladomiu,
and Josep Bassaganya-Riera*

Chapter 5 Ordinary Differential Equations (ODEs) Based Modeling...**63**

*Stefan Hoops, Raquel Hontecillas, Vida Abedi, Andrew Leber,
Casandra Philipson, Adria Carbo, and Josep Bassaganya-Riera*

*Vida Abedi, Stefan Hoops, Raquel Hontecillas, Adria Carbo,
Casandra Philipson, Monica Viladomiu, Andrew Leber,
Pinyi Lu, and Josep Bassaganya-Riera*

LIST OF CONTRIBUTORS

Vida Abedi
Nutritional Immunology and Molecular Medicine Laboratory, Virginia Bioinformatics Institute, Virginia Tech, Blacksburg, VA, USA

Maksudul Alam
Network Dynamics and Simulation Science Laboratory, Virginia Bioinformatics Institute, Virginia Tech, Blacksburg, VA, USA

Josep Bassaganya-Riera
Nutritional Immunology and Molecular Medicine Laboratory, Virginia Bioinformatics Institute, Virginia Tech, Blacksburg, VA, USA

Keith Bisset
Network Dynamics and Simulation Science Laboratory, Virginia Bioinformatics Institute, Virginia Tech, Blacksburg, VA, USA

Adria Carbo
Biotherapeutics Inc., Blacksburg, VA, USA

Xinwei Deng
Department of Statistics, Virginia Tech, Blacksburg, VA, USA

Stephen Eubank
Network Dynamics and Simulation Science Laboratory, Virginia Bioinformatics Institute, Virginia Tech, Blacksburg, VA, USA

Raquel Hontecillas
Nutritional Immunology and Molecular Medicine Laboratory, Virginia Bioinformatics Institute, Virginia Tech, Blacksburg, VA, USA

Stefan Hoops
Nutritional Immunology and Molecular Medicine Laboratory, Virginia Bioinformatics Institute, Virginia Tech, Blacksburg, VA, USA

Young Bun Kim
Nutritional Immunology and Molecular Medicine Laboratory, Virginia Bioinformatics Institute, Virginia Tech, Blacksburg, VA, USA

Barbara Kronsteiner
Nutritional Immunology and Molecular Medicine Laboratory, Virginia Bioinformatics Institute, Virginia Tech, Blacksburg, VA, USA

Andrew Leber
Nutritional Immunology and Molecular Medicine Laboratory, Virginia Bioinformatics Institute, Virginia Tech, Blacksburg, VA, USA

Pinyi Lu
Nutritional Immunology and Molecular Medicine Laboratory, Virginia Bioinformatics Institute, Virginia Tech, Blacksburg, VA, USA

Madhav Marathe
Network Dynamics and Simulation Science Laboratory, Virginia Bioinformatics Institute, Virginia Tech, Blacksburg, VA, USA

Pawel Michalak
Nutritional Immunology and Molecular Medicine Laboratory, Virginia Bioinformatics Institute, Virginia Tech, Blacksburg, VA, USA

Casandra Philipson
Biotherapeutics Inc., Blacksburg, VA, USA

Bruno W. Sobral
One Health Institute, Colorado State University, Fort Collins, CO, USA

Monica Viladomiu
Nutritional Immunology and Molecular Medicine Laboratory, Virginia Bioinformatics Institute, Virginia Tech, Blacksburg, VA, USA

Katherine Wendelsdorf
Applied Advanced Genomics, QIAGEN, Redwood City, CA, USA

CHAPTER *1*

Introduction to Computational Immunology

Josep Bassaganya-Riera and Raquel Hontecillas

Nutritional Immunology and Molecular Medicine Laboratory, Virginia Bioinformatics Institute, Virginia Tech, Blacksburg, VA, USA

OVERVIEW

The human immune system is a highly complex and dynamic self-organizing system that spans several orders of spatiotemporal magnitude critical for the maintenance of homeostasis and health. Traditional immunology research has generally employed reductionist approaches that evaluate in detail the individual components of the system disregarding that they are an integral part of a greater set of networks. This approach results in incremental knowledge discovery that fails to uncover complex, systems-wide mechanisms across scales or emerging context- and/or location-dependent behaviors. Computational modeling has revolutionized the study of immune responses as massively interacting information processing representations of the immune system, from molecules, to cells, to tissues, to systems and populations. To efficiently probe emerging and nonintuitive mechanisms of immune response, information processing representations of systems-wide interactions between cells, molecules, and microbiota components can be engineered by integrating diverse and big datasets, multiscale networks and, importantly, procedural knowledge through mathematical formalisms.

This book is based on notes, presentations, and other educational materials compiled during the Summer School and Symposium in Computational Immunology hosted by the Modeling Immunity to Enteric Pathogens (MIEP) at Virginia Tech (www.modelingimmunity. org) as well as research efforts undertaken as a part of this important NIAID-funded initiative. MIEP has pioneered the development of disruptive information biology technologies driven by high-performance computing (HPC), wet lab and *omic* data analytic

Computational Immunology: Models and Tools. DOI: http://dx.doi.org/10.1016/B978-0-12-803697-6.00001-1

capabilities, and large complex system modeling. MIEP's expertise is organized functionally to guide and underpin experimental research from computational hypothesis generation to data analytics, and from molecular science to accelerating the path to cures for widespread and debilitating human diseases, thereby accelerating the discovery and application of new knowledge. MIEP's cutting-edge immunoinformatics platform is enabled through newly developed information biology methodologies, including data analytics, modeling, and portal science.

MIEP's synthetic information biology technologies provide extreme scalability to support massively interacting systems such as complex host−pathogen−environment interactions and are currently able to support host response models with 10^7 to 10^{10} interacting elements. MIEP's information biology ecosystem integrates informatics, analytics, modeling with biological wet-lab sciences, and systems-wide analyses of host response to infection. This book describes in detail entirely new analytics and modeling technologies, and computer algorithms for studying mechanisms of immune response that inform the development of new classes of therapeutics.

When moving from traditional immunology research to the iterative systems immunology cycle, computer simulations guide and underpin experimental and clinical efforts, can advance the knowledge discovery cycle, and accelerate therapeutic development at an unprecedented rate. However, modeling complex systems such as the immune system requires multiscale modeling frameworks spanning from cells to systems and substantial computational resources. The latter is becoming especially accessible in todays' *Big Data* era. Biological systems are multiscale in nature, from molecules to tissues and from nanoseconds to a lifespan of several years. Hence, integration of multiple modeling technologies to understand immunological processes from signaling pathways within cells to lesion formation at the tissue level and toward clinical outcomes is the key to our understanding the complex system behavior and providing guidance for the modulation of the systems at multiple levels. This book summarizes the technical details of modeling targeted toward computational immunologists, bioinformaticians, and biologists. It reviews the latest cutting-edge implementation of modeling-enabled information biology.

MODELING TOOLS AND TECHNIQUES

Computational modeling techniques can capture existing procedural and mechanistic knowledge into models, combine theory with data, and discover new knowledge through model analyses and simulations. Emergence of computational biology [1] and modeling techniques [2,3] as well as the introduction of systems biology [4,5] have significantly influenced the developmental progress of computational tools and techniques. For instance, the rapid increase in computational power and accessibility to larger datasets were the driving force in the development and utilization of machine learning methodologies, statistical approaches, and methods from artificial intelligence applied to biological systems; furthermore, this trend is also favoring the development of novel techniques such as equation-free modeling for describing dynamic systems [6]. In addition, different fields have evolved in a unique way, in computational immunology, artificial immune systems [7,8] have emerged as an independent research area across multiple disciplines, including mathematics, engineering, computer science, and immunology.

In recent years, methods from artificial intelligence and machine learning have been applied and optimized for biological data with great success [9–17]. Statistical methods, including principal component analysis, partial least squares regression, partial least squares discriminant analysis, and Bayesian inference [18], have also significantly helped shape the data-driven modeling approaches. In addition, when mechanistic data is available for many entities for a given process, mechanistic model can also be constructed to further enhance our understanding of systems-level dynamics of the biological process. Equation-based models, captured using mathematical equations, such as ordinary differential equations (ODEs), difference equations, stochastic differential equations, and partial differential equations, can accurately capture quantitative changes of immunological markers in time and space. However, even though mathematical equations are often elegant and efficient representations, many biological phenomena cannot be easily captured using this formalism. Agent-based models (ABMs) can also be used to model interactions among various entities. ABM can help multiscale [19] and highly complex biological phenomena. These new modeling technologies are often computationally expensive and require deploying a cyberinfrastructure that provides linkages between modeling/simulation, clinical, and preclinical studies as well as the implementation in HPC settings (Chapter 4).

USE CASES ILLUSTRATING THE APPLICATION OF COMPUTATIONAL IMMUNOLOGY TECHNOLOGIES

Use Case 1: The development of gastritis during *Helicobacter pylori* infection is dependent on an activated adaptive immune response orchestrated by T helper (Th) cells [20–23]. However, the relative contributions of the Th1 and Th17 cell subsets to gastritis and control of infection are not fully elucidated. To investigate the role of interleukin-21 (IL-21) in the gastric mucosa during *H. pylori* infection, we combined mathematical modeling of CD4+ T-cell differentiation with *in vivo* mechanistic studies. Our deterministic and stochastic computational modeling results using our CD4+ T-cell differentiation model [24] revealed that the relative contributions of Th1 and Th17 are mediated through STAT1 and STAT3 mechanisms, respectively. The computational predictions also revealed that IL-21 has a key role in modulating IL-10 during gastritis in *H. pylori*-infected individuals. These predictions were fully validated using *in vivo* animal models of *H. pylori* infection, providing insight into a myriad of other infectious and immune disorders in which IL-21 is increasingly recognized to play a central role [25]. The use of IL-21-related therapies may provide treatment options for individuals chronically colonized with *H. pylori* as an alternative to aggressive antibiotics.

Use Case 2: Pattern-recognition receptors (PRRs) expressed by gastric epithelial cells and mucosal mononuclear phagocytes (MNPs; macrophages and dendritic cells) are essential for detecting *H. pylori* and govern subsequent effector and regulatory immune responses of innate and adaptive cells during infection [26]. *Helicobacter pylori* infection suppresses a unique subset of regulatory PRRs, including NLRX1, NLRP12, and NLRC3, in MNPs however limited mechanistic insight exists surrounding this phenomenon and its impact on dynamic regulation of inflammatory versus anti-inflammatory host responses, bacterial burden, and tissue damage at the gut mucosa [27]. To investigate the immunomodulatory roles of NLRX1, we engineered a deterministic ODE-based mathematical model based on network analysis of global gene expression for macrophages infected with *H. pylori* at six discrete time points. Our model simulates three spatiotemporal immune response waves that correlate to effector responses induced by extracellular and intracellular detection of *H. pylori* in addition to a novel regulatory element with robust transient behavior. The model predicts that NLRX1 is tightly regulated by early-induced regulatory molecules and is essential for *H. pylori* colonization. Through a series of follow-up experimental studies, we fully validate these model predictions and characterize a nonintuitive scenario for NLRX1 suppression. Taken together, this use case demonstrates how an iterative systems immunology cycle is applied to reveal novel broad-based mechanisms of mucosal immunity and host tolerance through computational and mathematical exploration of immunological feedback circuits.

Use Case 3: *Helicobacter pylori* is a dominant member of the human gastric microbiota that selectively establishes lifelong colonization of the gastric mucosa in over 50% of the human population [28,29]. Although *H. pylori* has been traditionally classified as a pathogen [30,31], most recent data suggests that persistent colonization could be responsible for protection against allergies, diabetes, asthma, and chronic inflammatory autoimmune diseases [32–37]. *Helicobacter pylori* infection of the gastric mucosa leads to induction of mixed effector and regulatory responses. However, these vigorous effector responses fail to rid host from the microorganism and *H. pylori* is able to persist chronically [38–46]. The immunoregulatory mechanisms for chronic microbial persistence and their implication in protective versus pathogenic outcomes of infection are incompletely understood. In this regard, we constructed tissue-level ODE-based and ABM computational and mathematical models of effector and regulatory mucosal immune responses to *H. pylori* [21,25], which identified macrophages as central regulators of chronic *H. pylori* colonization and gastric pathology. Interestingly, *in silico* shifting of macrophage phenotype into pro-inflammatory states resulted in decreased gastric microbial colonization and enhanced pathology. We successfully validated our computational predictions by experimentally depleting macrophages or shifting their phenotype into a pro-inflammatory state, which resulted in a 10-fold decrease in gastric bacterial loads. Moreover, we were able to identify an infiltrating IL-10-producing macrophage population essential for the induction of regulatory responses which facilitates colonization of the gastric niche. By combining computational and experimental efforts, we were able to effectively identify critical immunomodulators of

H. pylori infection, whose function could be exploited as tolerization strategies aiming to ameliorate not only *H. pylori*-related malignancies but also other extra-gastric disease conditions.

The following chapters provide an window to the use of modeling and simulation in modern immunology research by describing: the use of computational modeling approaches to accelerate immunology, infectious and immune-mediated disease research, the cyberinfrastructure required for computational modeling of immune responses, strategies to connect Big data, models, data and tools, ODE modeling, agent-based modeling, strategies multiscale modeling combining a variety of modeling technologies. Chapter 9 provides a series of real-life exercises that address important immunological questions by integrating the computational modeling knowledge presented in this book.

ACKNOWLEDGMENTS

This work was supported in part by National Institute of Allergy and Infectious Diseases Contract No. HHSN272201000056C to JBR and funds from the Nutritional Immunology and Molecular Medicine Laboratory (www.nimml.org).

REFERENCES

[1] Davison DB, et al. Whither computational biology. J Comput Biol 1994;1(1):1–2.

[2] Brown CT, et al. New computational approaches for analysis of cis-regulatory networks. Dev Biol 2002;246(1):86–102.

[3] Yuh CH, Bolouri H, Davidson EH. Genomic cis-regulatory logic: experimental and computational analysis of a sea urchin gene. Science 1998;279(5358):1896–902.

[4] Kitano H. Computational systems biology. Nature 2002;420(6912):206–10.

[5] Hucka M, et al. The systems biology markup language (SBML): a medium for representation and exchange of biochemical network models. Bioinformatics 2003;19(4):524–31.

[6] Ye H, et al. Equation-free mechanistic ecosystem forecasting using empirical dynamic modeling. Proc Natl Acad Sci USA 2015;112(13):E1569–76.

[7] Klarreich E. Inspired by immunity. Nature 2002;415(6871):468–70.

[8] Forrest S, Beauchemin C. Computer immunology. Immunol Rev 2007;216:176–97.

[9] Craven MW, Shavlik JW. Using neural networks for data mining. Future Generation Comp Syst 1997;13(2):211–29.

[10] Lu H, Setiono R, Liu H. Effective data mining using neural networks. IEEE Trans Knowl Data Eng 1996;8(6):957–61.

[11] Dayhoff JE, DeLeo JM. Artificial neural networks. Cancer 2001;91(S8):1615–35.

[12] Ling H, Samarasinghe S, Kulasiri D. Novel recurrent neural network for modelling biological networks: oscillatory p53 interaction dynamics. Biosystems 2013;114(3):191−205.

[13] Snow PB, Smith DS, Catalona WJ. Artificial neural networks in the diagnosis and prognosis of prostate cancer: a pilot study. J Urol 1994;152(5 Pt 2):1923−6.

[14] Lek S, Guégan J-F. Artificial neural networks as a tool in ecological modelling, an introduction. Ecol Modell 1999;120(2):65−73.

[15] Brusic V, Rudy G, Harrison LC. Prediction of MHC binding peptides using artificial neural networks. Complex Syst: Mech Adaptation 1994:253−60.

[16] Lu P, Abedi V, Mei Y, Hontecillas R, Philipson C, Hoops S, et al. Supervised learning with artificial neural network in modeling of cell differentiation process. In: Tran QN, Arabnia H, editors. Emerging trends in computational biology, bioinformatics, and systems biology. 1st ed. Burlington, Massachusetts: Morgan Kaufmann; 2015. p. 1−18.

[17] Lu P, et al. Supervised learning methods in modeling of CD4+ T cell heterogeneity. BioData Min 2015;8:27.

[18] Benedict KF, Lauffenburger DA. Insights into proteomic immune cell signaling and communication via data-driven modeling. Curr Top Microbiol Immunol 2013;363:201−33.

[19] Mei Y, et al. Multiscale modeling of mucosal immune responses. BMC Bioinformatics 2015;16(Suppl. 12):S2.

[20] Algood HM, et al. Host response to Helicobacter pylori infection before initiation of the adaptive immune response. FEMS Immunol Med Microbiol 2007;51(3):577−86.

[21] Carbo A, et al. Predictive computational modeling of the mucosal immune responses during Helicobacter pylori infection. PLoS One 2013;8(9):e73365.

[22] Karttunen R, et al. Interferon gamma and interleukin 4 secreting cells in the gastric antrum in Helicobacter pylori positive and negative gastritis. Gut 1995;36(3):341−5.

[23] Bamford KB, et al. Lymphocytes in the human gastric mucosa during Helicobacter pylori have a T helper cell 1 phenotype. Gastroenterology 1998;114(3):482−92.

[24] Carbo A, et al. Systems modeling of molecular mechanisms controlling cytokine-driven CD4+ T cell differentiation and phenotype plasticity. PLoS Comput Biol 2013;9(4): e1003027.

[25] Carbo A, et al. Systems modeling of the role of interleukin-21 in the maintenance of effector CD4+ T cell responses during chronic Helicobacter pylori infection. MBio 2014;5(4): e01243−14

[26] Muller A, Oertli M, Arnold IC. H. pylori exploits and manipulates innate and adaptive immune cell signaling pathways to establish persistent infection. Cell Commun Signal 2011; 9(1):25.

[27] Castano-Rodriguez N, et al. The NOD-like receptor signalling pathway in Helicobacter pylori infection and related gastric cancer: a case-control study and gene expression analyses. PLoS One 2014;9(6):e98899.

[28] Stolte M. Helicobacter pylori gastritis and gastric MALT-lymphoma. Lancet 1992;339 (8795):745−6.

[29] Pernitzsch SR, Sharma CM. Transcriptome complexity and riboregulation in the human pathogen Helicobacter pylori. Front Cell Infect Microbiol 2012;2:14.

[30] Suerbaum S, Michetti P. Helicobacter pylori infection. N Engl J Med 2002;347(15):1175−86.

[31] Amieva MR, El-Omar EM. Host−bacterial interactions in Helicobacter pylori infection. Gastroenterology 2008;134(1):306−23.

[32] Pacifico L, et al. Consequences of Helicobacter pylori infection in children. World J Gastroenterol 2010;16(41):5181−94.

[33] Arnold IC, et al. *Helicobacter pylori* infection prevents allergic asthma in mouse models through the induction of regulatory T cells. J Clin Invest 2011;121(8):3088–93.

[34] Selgrad M, et al. *Helicobacter pylori* but not gastrin is associated with the development of colonic neoplasms. Int J Cancer 2014;135(5):1127–31.

[35] Bassaganya-Riera J, et al. *Helicobacter pylori* colonization ameliorates glucose homeostasis in mice through a PPAR gamma-dependent mechanism. PLoS One 2012;7(11):e50069.

[36] Cook KW, et al. *Helicobacter pylori* infection reduces disease severity in an experimental model of multiple sclerosis. Front Microbiol 2015;6:52.

[37] Engler DB, et al. Effective treatment of allergic airway inflammation with *Helicobacter pylori* immunomodulators requires BATF3-dependent dendritic cells and IL-10. Proc Natl Acad Sci USA 2014;111(32):11810–15.

[38] Lundgren A, et al. *Helicobacter pylori*-specific CD4+ CD25 high regulatory T cells suppress memory T-cell responses to *H. pylori* in infected individuals. Infect Immun 2003;71 (4):1755–62.

[39] Raghavan S, Suri-Payer E, Holmgren J. Antigen-specific *in vitro* suppression of murine *Helicobacter pylori*-reactive immunopathological T cells by CD4CD25 regulatory T cells. Scand J Immunol 2004;60(1–2):82–8.

[40] Rad R, et al. CD25+/Foxp3+ T cells regulate gastric inflammation and *Helicobacter pylori* colonization *in vivo*. Gastroenterology 2006;131(2):525–37.

[41] Lundgren A, et al. Mucosal FOXP3-expressing CD4+ CD25 high regulatory T cells in *Helicobacter pylori*-infected patients. Infect Immun 2005;73(1):523–31.

[42] Kandulski A, et al. Naturally occurring regulatory T cells (CD4+, CD25 high, FOXP3+) in the antrum and cardia are associated with higher *H. pylori* colonization and increased gene expression of TGF-beta1. Helicobacter 2008;13(4):295–303.

[43] Harris PR, et al. *Helicobacter pylori* gastritis in children is associated with a regulatory T-cell response. Gastroenterology 2008;134(2):491–9.

[44] Kao JY, et al. *Helicobacter pylori* immune escape is mediated by dendritic cell-induced Treg skewing and Th17 suppression in mice. Gastroenterology 2010;138(3):1046–54.

[45] Kao JY, et al. *Helicobacter pylori*-secreted factors inhibit dendritic cell IL-12 secretion: a mechanism of ineffective host defense. Am J Physiol Gastrointest Liver Physiol 2006;291(1): G73–81.

[46] Bimczok D, et al. Human primary gastric dendritic cells induce a Th1 response to *H. pylori*. Mucosal Immunol 2010;3(3):260–9.

CHAPTER 2

Computational Modeling

Josep Bassaganya-Riera[1], Raquel Hontecillas[1], Vida Abedi[1],
Adria Carbo[2], Casandra Philipson[2], and Stefan Hoops[1]

[1]Nutritional Immunology and Molecular Medicine Laboratory, Virginia Bioinformatics Institute,
Virginia Tech, Blacksburg, VA, USA [2]Biotherapeutics Inc., Blacksburg, VA, USA

OVERVIEW ON COMPUTATIONAL MODELING

The immune system is complex, ever evolving, dynamic, and self-organizing and plays a crucial role in the maintenance of health and prevention of disease. Comprehensively understanding its properties and function requires forming a coherent picture of the interplay between inflammatory and regulatory responses from molecules and cells to systems. Traditional immunology research has generally focused on the individual components of the immune system while disregarding their role as interconnected entities in a greater network. Computational modeling is revolutionizing the study of immune responses as massively interacting information processing representations of the immune system. The space of possible immunological mechanisms and new therapeutic pathways is enormous. It is not feasible to explore this space adequately through *in vivo* and *in vitro* experimentation (preclinical or clinical) alone. Mathematical models are being used to efficiently guide experimental designs that will most efficiently narrow the range of mechanisms to be explored. These models should be able to determine, for example, those time points at which data will best distinguish between alternative hypotheses concerning the time course of a mucosal or systemic immune response. Models should also allow us to generalize from *in vitro* results to *in vivo*, from wild-type mice to knockouts systems, from one animal model to another, and ultimately from animal models to human translation so that the most new knowledge is gained with the fewest resources spent.

Computational Immunology: Models and Tools. DOI: http://dx.doi.org/10.1016/B978-0-12-803697-6.00002-3

To efficiently probe emerging and unintuitive mechanisms of immune response, information processing representations of systems-wide interactions between cells, molecules, tissues, and microbiota components can be engineered *in silico* by integrating diverse and big datasets, multiscale networks and, importantly, procedural knowledge through mathematical formalisms. Since the immune system is inherently a multiscale system, modeling immune responses requires using multiple modeling technologies, multiscalability, collecting data from several sources such as public data repositories as well as collecting "model adequate" time course data from new experiments, collecting theory and procedural knowledge from the literature, and leveraging curated cellular and molecular networks.

MIEP's information biology technologies have centered on how modeling, data analytics, and portal science work together to engineer large-scale synthetic immune systems. However, the complex, multiscale nature of the immune system means that the mathematical models will not be amenable to an analytic solution. Hence computational simulations of the models are necessary. In order to effectively guide experimental design, computational models must capture multiple kinds of dynamics at multiple scales within the system. There are several established methods, such as hybrid agent-based model (ABM) or particle-in-a-cell, for representing different dynamics at different scales within a single computation. These methods are based on assumptions about separation-of-scale, such as slow versus fast dynamics. There is no framework that makes it easy to explore the implications of a particular set of assumptions about scale in a biological, especially immunological, context.

MIEP provides a novel conceptual framework pioneering the use of multiscale modeling in immunology and infectious disease research (see Chapter 8). Although many computational modeling techniques have been used in immunology [1–3], ours was the first group to publish a computational model for gastrointestinal immunity [4]. MIEP's models of the mucosal immune system capture responses to infection occurring across multiple spatiotemporal and organizational scales from the intracellular signaling to the tissue-level responses and lesion formation. Indeed, *Helicobacter pylori* infection represents an ideal model system to study immune response dynamics leading to disease versus beneficial health outcomes.

TRANSLATIONAL RESEARCH ITERATIVE MODELING CYCLE

This chapter uses the example of modeling immune responses to describe the nuts and bolts of applying the computational modeling process to accelerate systems immunology and infectious disease research.

Computational modeling requires articulating the model building process around a scientific problem or a question that cannot be addressed through traditional experimental approaches generally due to the large scope. The modeling exercise is inherently transdisciplinary given that it transcends each of the disciplines that allow it to happen and it is articulated as a problem-solving activity. For instance, modeling immune responses requires the participation of teams of individuals with expertise in immunology, mathematics, computer science, high-performance computing, engineering, and bioinformatics. While the initial questions to be addressed are immunological in nature, the products derived from modeling are broadly applicable to other disciplines such as biological metaphors that inform the design of next-generation computational systems. For newly established modeling teams, the first step of the process should be to align the semantics among team members with diverse training and expertise and make sure that immunologists understand the language of computer scientists and vice versa. Following this initial phase, frequent transdisciplinary team meetings focused around developing models are needed to maintain the momentum.

The modeling process that enables the translational information biology cycle is subdivided into the following steps, which are illustrated in Figure 2.1 and further described below:

 I. Knowledge extraction from literature
 II. Collect new data generation and data from public repositories
 III. Network model development
 IV. *In silico* experimentation
 V. Computational hypothesis testing and *in vivo/in vitro* validation.

The steps of this cycle require iteration and are found at the core of translational systems biology research.

INFORMATION AND KNOWLEDGE EXTRACTION FROM THE LITERATURE

Effective literature search and exploration is necessary for accurate model development and it can lead to novel hypothesis generation.

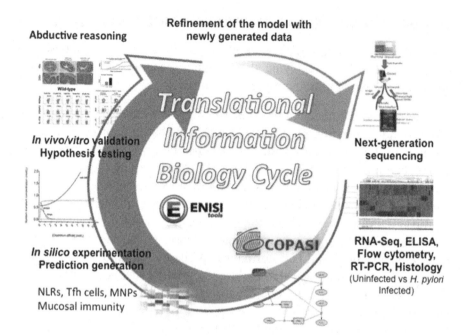

Figure 2.1 Integrated and iterative modeling pipeline.

However, with the exponential growth in the number of scientific journals and papers it is unfeasible to manually scan the literature. For instance, PubMed with over 24 million citations (and increasing roughly 30,000 per day) is searched over 6 million times on an average daily basis. To effectively reduce information overload, it is imperative to explore and utilize novel tools (see Refs. [5,6–18]) that are being developed to accelerate knowledge discovery, promote interdisciplinary collaboration, and serve the scientific community at large.

Tools and state-of-the-art technologies can not only help in filtering information and summarizing text, but also facilitate discover new knowledge. For instance, we have recently developed a large-scale literature-mining tool ARIANA+ (Adaptive Robust and Integrative Analysis for finding Novel Associations) capable of capturing direct and indirect associations among 2545 biomedical concepts [6–9]. Tools such as ARIANA+ are specifically suited for biomedical applications because they can be customized to include the rich context specific terminology; in fact, it is estimated that medical records in pathology can include over 12,000 medical abbreviations [19].

In addition, the scientific vocabulary is also dynamic. This is to highlight the challenges in developing robust, scalable, and context-specific tools that can address the specific needs of the scientific community.

In addition to text-mining tools and technologies, there are also curated knowledge base repositories [20–22] that are being developed and maintained to facilitate knowledge discovery and enable strategic reading and filtering of information. These databases provide also visualization capabilities that can aid in knowledge representation and extraction.

Exploratory   Research   in   Immunology   Using   ARIANA+: *Helicobacter pylori* is a Gram-negative bacteria that chronically persists in 50% of the human population and in 15% of the infected people it causes serious pathologies like gastric ulcer. Using the tool to perform a global literature search with *"Helicobacter pylori"* as keyword brings out interesting associations. The top three associated headings are: (1) *Lipoproteins > Apolipoproteins > Apolipoproteins B*; (2) *Physiological Effects of Drugs > Neurotransmitter Agents > Adrenergic   Agents >   Adrenergic   Agonists >   Adrenergic   alpha-Agonists*; and (3) *Isonicotinic Acids*. In the second category of associated entities, we extract 14 additional headings that might have potential associations with *H. pylori* (Table 2.1). Among these "Diabetes Mellitus, Type 1" and "diabetic angi-opathies" are of special interest. *Helicobacter pylori* commensalism has been linked with amelioration of Diabetes Mellitus Type II (T2DM) [27]; among the 2545 Medical Subject Headings that are part of the model in ARIANA+ system includes "Diabetes Mellitus, Type I," "Gestational Diabetes" as well as "Diabetic Angiopathies." Diabetes Mellitus, Type II is not included in the model as it was associated with a very large body of literature. However, detecting Type I Diabetes as well as diabetic angiopathies as potentially associated entities is an important indication of potential link between T2DM and *H. pylori*. Further global literature search was performed to verify whether diabetes is associated with inflammatory bowel disease (IBD) and/or Gram-negative bacterial infections. A search for "diabetes" using ARIANA+ returns 60 highly associated entities and 106 possibly associated entities and interestingly IBD as well as Gram-negative bacterial infection are among the results, thus further corroborating the association between *H. pylori* and diabetes.

Table 2.1 Top Ranked Headings and Their Score Measure with Respect to "*Helicobacter pylori*"

Associated Medical Subject Headings (MeSH)	Score
Lipoproteins > Apolipoproteins > Apolipoproteins B	High
Physiological Effects of Drugs > Neurotransmitter Agents > Adrenergic Agents > Adrenergic Agonists > **Adrenergic alpha-Agonists**	High
Isonicotinic Acids	High
Oral Fistula	Medium
Identification (Psychology) > **Gender Identity**	Medium
Urogenital Abnormalities > **Urinary Fistula**	Medium
Fistula > **Urinary Fistula**	Medium
Leishmaniasis > **Leishmaniasis, Cutaneous**	Medium
Encephalomyelitis	Medium
Death > **Fetal Death**	Medium
Lip Diseases	Medium
Stomatognathic System Abnormalities > Maxillofacial Abnormalities > **Jaw Abnormalities**	Medium
Sexuality > **Homosexuality**	Medium
Skin Manifestations > Purpura > **Purpura, Thrombocytopenic**	Medium
Glucose Metabolism Disorders > Diabetes Mellitus > Diabetes Mellitus, Type 1	Medium
Diabetic Angiopathies	Medium
Sarcoma, Experimental	Medium

COLLECT NEW DATA AND DATA FROM PUBLIC REPOSITORIES

The modeling process requires *in vitro*, preclinical, mechanistic, and clinical data to build predictive computational models. More importantly, modeling shapes how the data are collected. For instance, given cost considerations, detailed time-course series data with seven or more time points are rarely collected in the context of traditional immunology experimentation. However, to accurately represent the dynamics and evolution of immune responses and how the immune system responds to therapeutic interventions and vaccines, time-course studies are necessary. The database that is used to train the model to behave like the biological system being studied is called calibration database. Such database can be build based on data from the literature, data repositories such as GEO, ImmPort, etc. (see Chapter 4 for more information) or in some cases when the key data needed for model calibration is not available, then designing experiments for collecting the calibration dataset is required. Examples of calibration data types for building computational models of the immune response include RNA-seq, RT-PCR, flow cytometry, CYTOF, ELISA, histology and immunohistochemistry images, pathogen burden, and composition of microbiota interacting with the host. These calibration datasets generally end up as supplementary information in computational immunology publications [23–25]. Chapter 9 provides some examples of calibration datasets and how these datasets can be used to train the computational models. Modeling-derived computational hypothesis require experimental validation. The experimental data collected to validate a modeling prediction can become a calibration dataset in the next iteration of the modeling cycle.

MODEL DEVELOPMENT

Modeling immunity encompasses intracellular, cellular, and tissue-level scales. Complex biological relationships among species of distinct scales defined in our models are represented as networks using CellDesigner software. The network architecture is developed based on experimental data generated by our team, comprehensive literature searches, data mining public repositories, for example, Gene expression omnibus [26], ImmPort. *Modeling* intimately links network inference methods with literature searches in order to: (1) quickly identify high-priority molecules and canonical signaling cascades based on time and treatment of samples; (2) ensure accuracy of predicted reactions from network inference and analyses methods and highly curated knowledge base; and (3) allow easy customization of molecular networks based on hypotheses and calibration datasets.

Our models contain a broad array of biological processes including ligand–receptor binding, protein–protein interactions, transport between compartments, transcription, translation, and degradation. Three kinetic equations are commissioned for computational modeling of such biological processes, namely: (1) mass action, (2) Michaelis–Menten, and (3) Hill equation kinetics [27]. Additionally, dynamic behavior of biological networks often contains reoccurring wiring patterns known as "network motifs" that must be taken into consideration mathematically. One of the most integral network motifs is the feed-forward loop (FFL) that occurs during molecular cross talk [28]; for instance, molecule A regulates molecule B yet molecules A and B coregulate molecule C. FFLs are undoubtedly a common theme in our models and thus mathematics underlying macrophage signaling networks will adopt a combination of equations and parameters as justified herein.

The Hill equation is a sigmoidal function that easily represents switch mechanisms, such as transcription factor binding. The Hill model provides an advantage for estimating in a precise fashion to what extent positive or negative cooperativity between molecules exists [27]. Extensive studies have also demonstrated the benefits of the Hill equation for studying combinatorial regulation, especially those observed in FFLs [29], and therefore Hill equations will be used initially for characterizing cooperative roles among nod-like receptors (NLRs). Additionally, molecules that are regulated by several inputs (i.e., one gene jointly regulated by two transcription factors) may be calibrated given the assignment of a Hill equation.

Mass action equations provide some advantages over Hill equations primarily related to their inherent ability to decipher mechanisms underlying molecular cooperativity rather than just positive or negative regulation (Hill model) [27]. Degradation rates and molecule transport are accurately represented by mass action equations. Mass action kinetics are also suitable for modeling multisite protein phosphorylation and will be implemented in our studies due to their reliability in deterministic and stochastic simulations [30–32]. We will also consider implementing mass action equations for transcription and combinatorial regulation reactions in models used for stochastic simulations.

Parameter estimation will be performed on unknown constant values using the Genetic Algorithm and Particle Swarm algorithms in COPASI. Numerical boundaries will be applied such that reaction rates are estimated in a biologically relevant range (e.g., transcription factor mRNA decay rates could be given a parameter search space of 1–3 h [33]). Fitting results will be thoroughly analyzed using COPASI's objective functions results and cross-referenced to experimental data for calculating standard error [24]. Models deemed calibrated by these standards will then be used for *in silico* experimentation outlined below.

Further details on the optimal functions to be used for each type of reactions and how to parameterize and calibrate the models based on experimental data will be provided in examples of Chapter 9.

IN SILICO EXPERIMENTATION

In silico experimentation involves performing perturbations to the calibrated model to determine how changes in one or more species or agents influence the entire *in silico* immune system. Such perturbations can range from infection with an organism, depletion of cell subset, and creation of an *in silico* knockout. Furthermore, even though *in silico* experimentation has been used extensively and been successful in hypothesis generation, there is still lack of confidence in the reliability and robustness as well as applicability of the models. To address these concerns, different studies (such as Ref. [34]) have proposed assessment schemes for the scientific validity of the models in accordance with the principles of modeling practices. However, modeling and simulation are increasingly being explored in a unified manner and their success has been the driving force toward novel and nonintuitive experimentation. Furthermore, using *in silico* experimentation it is possible to enhance the quality of care by performing patient stratification and dose selection. Such studies can be performed by using virtual clinical population [35]. A virtual population that is designed to mimic characteristics and features of the real population can be very useful in identifying key elements of the condition. Finally, a very important tool for *in silico* experimentation is the sensitivity analyses (SAs). For instance, using SA on virtual clinical trial simulation, it was possible to identify least and most important parameters that could affect the clinical outcome. For instance, the results of the study indicated that inhibition of IL-6 produced a small survival benefit while inhibition of IL1β did not significantly affect the outcome.

Parameter sensitivity comprises two different questions: (1) the sensitivity of the model (or parts thereof) to changes of a parameter and (2) the sensitivity of the parameters to collected experimental values.

The first question addresses the sensitivity of the model to parameter changes is routinely addressed during our modeling process. For example, even before parameters are known we use global parameter sensitivity as described in Ref. [36] to determine which parameters do not affect the model thus reducing the number of parameters to be estimated during the fitting process. The global SA is performed using Condor-COPASI [37]. Once the model is calibrated, we use local sensitivities that can be performed in COPASI directly to determine the effect on the model of the parameters. It is possible in COPASI (or Condor-COPASI) to specify any observable or a mathematical expression of multiple observables (e.g., ratio of pro-inflammatory cytokine vs anti-inflammatory) at as the effect to be caused by a parameter change. Thus, SA in COPASI is a very powerful to determine the main parameters which influence the health outcome.

We have developed a similar approach as described in Ref. [36] for the ABMs. In a paper under development, we describe a statistical approach that analyzes the effect of any pairwise parameter changes. Careful experimental design allows us to avoid simulating the model for a wide range of parameter values and all pairwise combinations. This experimental design is required since it is computationally not feasible to simulate ABM (or multiscale models) thousands of times. Quantifying the impact of parameter uncertainty in large and complex ABMs is very challenging due to the large number of parameters and the associated computational cost. We have developed a SA framework to address the sensitivity of the parameters at the global and local scales (paper in development). The global scale measures the significance of each parameter while the local scale measures the local effect of different parameters. Our method efficiently identifies the most significant parameters and unveils their contributions to the outcomes of the system. To address the SA in ABM, we are using the ENteric Immunity SImulator (ENISI) as a modeling environment for studying the inflammatory/effector and regulatory immune responses in the gut. In essence, SA for ABMs enhances the understanding of the influence of different input parameters and their variations on the model outcomes. SA is also important for understanding the relationships between input and output variables, testing the robustness of the system, and identifying the errors in the model. This framework is described in Chapter 8.

VALIDATION OF COMPUTATIONAL HYPOTHESES AND NEW KNOWLEDGE

This is the most critical step of the entire modeling process since the results of validation experiments designed with the guidance of the previous modeling steps validate or invalidate the computational hypotheses. This step is not much different than traditional immunology experimentation with one major caveat: in traditional immunology the decisions on experimental design are based on the synthesis of information in the brains of an individual or a team, whereas in modeling the previous information, data and knowledge has been integrated and synthesized *in silico* and decisions are supported by data analytics and visualization tools.

All modeling assumptions are made in collaboration between modelers and the experimental and immunology domain experts. In fact, modeling and experimentation are advising each other. In a circular process, experimental results are used to refine and enhance the models. The enhanced model is analyzed and investigated for interesting and novel results, which than are attempted to be validated by the experimental team. If the predictions are validated the resulting data is used to improve the model parameter. If, however, the predictions cannot be validated the result can still be used to modify the model parameters so that the experimentally observed behavior is captured by the model. Should the modification of the parameters not correct the model behavior, we will modify the model network topology with the help of the experimenters and immunology domain experts. Once this is achieved, the cycle starts anew. This process assures that the model addresses the observed biology. We have used this systems immunology cycle successfully to build several models in MIEP [23−25,38−43].

Calibrating the complex models of immune response requires a careful model verification process [44]. However, multiscale models of immune responses have a large input parameter space and high-dimensional output space. Investigating all possible settings for model verification is not practical. Thus, in that context one can utilize a sequential and adaptive model verification strategy under the concept of information-oriented design of experiments. The proposed strategy enables the efficient reduction of the number of search iterations to achieve optimal calibration. Specifically, the objective is to find an optimal set of input parameters with small iteration steps. We first conduct a space-filling sampling [45,46] of parameters to carve out the noninformative regions of the parameter space. Then we apply factor screening in experimental design [47,48] to identify the significant parameters. Finally, the adaptive response surface method is used to seek the sets of parameter values that result in the best-performing simulation outputs. Nonlinear optimization tools will be used to facilitate the search for optimal parameters [49,50] in the adaptive response surface method.

CONSIDERATIONS ON COMPUTATIONAL MODELING TECHNOLOGIES

As described in Chapter 1, computational modeling techniques can capture existing knowledge into models and discover new knowledge through model analyses and simulations. Methods from artificial intelligence and machine learning have been applied and optimized for biological data with great success [51–59]. Statistical methods, including principal component analysis, partial least squares regression, partial least squares discriminant analysis, and Bayesian inference [60], have also significantly helped shape the data-driven modeling approaches. The causal, explanatory models we have built represent the interactions of discrete entities such as molecules, cells, tissues, and organs. If the interactions are nonlinear, or the sets of entities that interact are not well mixed, then an ABM is an appropriate representation (see Chapter 6 for further details on ABM). However, at very small or very large spatial scales, or if the experimental protocol does not control for the mixing rate, the results will not be sensitive to the lack of mixing. In this situation, representation as a set of differential equations is appropriate. If spatial heterogeneity is important, the differential equations will include spatial derivatives and thus become partial differential equations (PDEs); if spatial heterogeneity can be ignored and the discrete nature of the entities is not important, ordinary differential equation (ODE) models are sufficiently powerful (described in detail in Chapter 5). If the discrete nature of the entities is important, then regardless of all the other considerations, ABMs are again a natural representation. Finally, if random fluctuations are important, such as in processes controlled by lowly expressed RNA then stochasticity must be introduced into each of these modeling approaches. The next section describes the user-friendly tools that enable these distinct types of modeling immune responses.

COMPUTATIONAL MODELING TOOLS FOR IMMUNOLOGY AND INFECTIOUS DISEASE RESEARCH

The emergence of computational biology [61] and modeling techniques [62,63] as well as the introduction of systems biology [64,65] has significantly influenced the developmental progress of computational tools and techniques. Some of the user-friendly tools used for immune modeling are described below.

COPASI: COPASI [66,67] is a software application for simulation and analysis of biochemical networks and their dynamics. It is a stand-alone program which supports models in the SBML standard and enables simulating their behaviors based on ODEs or stochastic simulation algorithms based on the work of Gillespie [68,69]. COPASI is equipped with extensive support for parameter estimation, SA, stability analysis optimization, and output visualization. It is used in many areas of biomedical research, including drug design [70], cancer modeling [71,72], neurochemistry [73–75], environmental health [76], immunology [77,78], metabolism [79,80], biotechnology [81,82], and origin of life studies [83]. We plan to implement a new algorithm called stochastic differential equations (SDEs) in COPASI. SDE for stochastic modeling has been widely used for economics and statistics [84]. However, only a few studies [85–89] apply SDE in computational biology modeling. In terms of SDE modeling tools, we have found one SDE package in Matlab and one in R [84]; however, they are difficult to use. Implementing SDE in COPASI will for the first time provide a user-friendly SDE modeling tool and greatly increase the system-level stochastic modeling capability for computational biology.

ENISI: As a part of MIEP project, we have developed ENISI, a modeling system for inflammatory and regulatory immune pathways initiated by microbe–immune cell interactions in the gut. ENISI is an interaction-based model in which individual cells and cell–cell interactions are modeled probabilistically. ENISI has the ability to simulate at least 10^7 individual cells. With ENISI, immunologists are able to test and generate hypotheses for enteric disease pathology and propose interventions through experimental infection of an *in silico* gut. Simulation outcomes under different experimental conditions allow observation of *in silico* behaviors that are not readily seen through *in vitro* and *in vivo* techniques. The ENISI modeling environment has already been illustrated by developing (i) an *in silico* model and dynamic simulation of *H. pylori* [90,91] and (ii) a simulation of dysentery resulting from *Brachyspira hyodysenteriae* infection [91] so as to identify aspects of the host responses that lead to immune tissue damage even after pathogen clearance.

ENISI Visual [92] (Figure 2.2) is an ABM tool for simulating immune responses to enteric pathogens. It was developed based upon Repast Simphony [93], a popular ABM platform. It has three

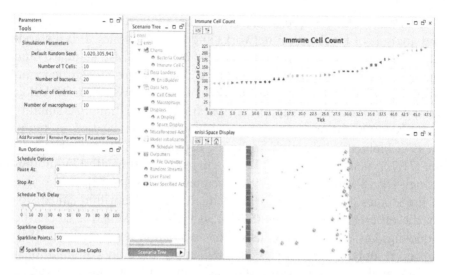

Figure 2.2 ENISI User Interface. Users can specify initial cell and pathogen concentrations, simulation speed, output charts, figures, and videos.

compartments: lumen, epithelial, and lamina propia and simulates seven types of cells including epithelial cells, T cells, B cells, macrophages, neutrophils, dendritic cells, and bacteria. Each cell type can have several subtypes. For example, T cells can be resting T cells, T Helper cells, or T regulatory cells.

ENISI Visual is adapted from the HPC implementations of ENISI and emphasizes quality user interfaces and visualizations. ENISI Visual allows users to specify the initial concentrations of cells, the pathogen infectious dose, and simulation time. From the interface, users can control the animation speed and specify the output charts, figures, real-time animations, snapshots, and videos. ENISI Visual has integrated secretion and propagation of cytokines and chemokines, and the cell movement models.

ENISI SDE. SDE modeling has been widely used in economics and statistics [19]. However, only a few studies [85–89] applied SDE into computational biology modeling. For those studies, the models are relatively small in scale with only a few ODEs and some of them used Matlab to directly build the SDEs. We have found one SDE package in Matlab [35] and one in R [19]; however, they are not user-friendly, especially when biologists with limited computational training want to use them. While deterministic modeling strategies are widely used in computational biology, stochastic modeling techniques are not as popular due to a lack of user-friendly tools. This chapter presents ENISI SDE, a novel web-based modeling tool with SDEs. ENISI SDE provides user-friendly web user interfaces to facilitate adoption by immunologists and computational biologists. We developed ENISI SDE as a web-based user-friendly SDE modeling tool that highly resembles regular ODE-based modeling. Under MIEP we applied SDE modeling tool through as use case for studying stochastic sources of cell heterogeneity in the context of the CD4+ T-cell differentiation. The case study clearly shows the effectiveness of SDE as a stochastic modeling approach in biology in general and immunology in particular and the power of ENISI SDE [94].

ENISI MSM is a platform developed under MIEP that integrates ENISI Visual and COPASI [66]. ENISI MSM is designed for the simulation of multiscale models covering intracellular, intercellular, and tissue-level scales. Component wise, an ENISI MSM model can cover signaling pathways, metabolic networks, gene-regulatory networks, cytokine and chemokine diffusions, cell movement, and tissue compartments at the same time (Figure 2.3).

ENISI MSM is a prototype of a multiscale modeling tool, which integrates ABMs, ODE models, and PDE models to represent the dynamics of gut mucosal immunity from intracellular to tissue scales in the gastrointestinal mucosa.

The development of a multiscale model that encompasses intracellular signaling pathways, cell—cell interactions, cognate versus non-cognate interactions in a healthy versus diseased gastric mucosa is highly innovative. ENISI MSM combines four orders of spatiotemporal magnitude [95]. Distinct spatiotemporal scales have different properties requiring diverse modeling techniques. The use of ODE and SDE to model intracellular signaling pathways, in combination with PDEs to simulate cytokine/chemokine diffusions and cell movement, and ABM for cell—cell interactions at the cellular and population level, integrates all four spatiotemporal scales together with a unique multi-simulation platform: ENISI. In sum, utilizing an innovative multiscale modeling approach, this project will conceptualize the effects of targeted molecular perturbation on whole tissue pathology during infection (Figure 2.3). Our ABMs are built on rigorous mathematical foundations—one of the unique aspects of our work called Graphical

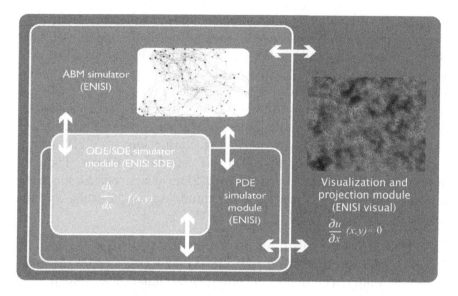

Figure 2.3 Software architecture of the ENISI MSM tool.

Discrete Dynamical Systems [96,97], which have been used to build ENISI, a tool capable of MSM at unprecedented scales of 10^7 to 10^{10} agents [98]. Further details on multiscale modeling are provided in Chapter 8.

CONCLUDING REMARKS

Under MIEP we have articulated a highly synergistic paradigm-shifting computational modeling strategy for characterizing mechanisms of immunoregulation in infectious and immune-mediated diseases spanning several orders of spatiotemporal magnitude. The user-friendly modeling tools and scalable models developed represent information processing representations of massively interacting immune response. Connecting models, data, and tools to build such scalable models requires a substantial immunoinformatics cyberinfrastructure that is described in detail throughout Chapters 4 and 7.

ACKNOWLEDGMENTS

This work was supported in part by National Institute of Allergy and Infectious Diseases Contract No. HHSN272201000056C to JBR and funds from the Nutritional Immunology and Molecular Medicine Laboratory (www.nimml.org).

REFERENCES

[1] Kirschner D, Panetta JC. Modeling immunotherapy of the tumor–immune interaction. J Math Biol 1998;37(3):235–52.

[2] Wigginton JE, Kirschner D. A model to predict cell-mediated immune regulatory mechanisms during human infection with *Mycobacterium tuberculosis*. J Immunol 2001;166(3): 1951–67.

[3] Marino S, et al. A methodology for performing global uncertainty and sensitivity analysis in systems biology. J Theor Biol 2008;254(1):178–96.

[4] Wendelsdorf K, et al. Model of colonic inflammation: immune modulatory mechanisms in inflammatory bowel disease. J Theor Biol 2010;264(4):1225–39.

[5] Lu Z. PubMed and beyond: a survey of web tools for searching biomedical literature. Database: J Biol Databases Curation 2011;2011:baq036.

[6] Abedi V, Yeasin M, Zand R. Empirical study using network of semantically related associations in bridging the knowledge gap. J Transl Med 2014;12:324.

[7] Abedi V, et al. An automated framework for hypotheses generation using literature. BioData Min 2012;5:13.

[8] Abedi V, Yeasin M, Zand R. ARIANA: adaptive robust and integrative analysis for finding novel associations. The 2014 international conference on advances in big data analytics. Las Vegas, NV: CSREA Press; 2014. p. 22–8.

[9] Abedi V, Yeasin M, Zand R. Literature mining and ontology mapping applied to big data. In: Akhgar B, Saathoff G, Arabnia H, Hill R, Staniforth A, Bayerl, editors. Mining big data to improve national security. Waltham, MA: Elsevier; 2015. p. 184–208.

[10] Rzhetsky A, Seringhaus M, Gerstein M. Seeking a new biology through text mining. Cell 2008;134:9–13.

[11] Mishra R, et al. Text summarization in the biomedical domain: a systematic review of recent research. J Biomed Inform 2014.

[12] Verspoor KM. Roles for text mining in protein function prediction. Methods Mol Biol 2014;1159:95–108.

[13] Wei C-H, et al. Accelerating literature curation with text-mining tools: a case study of using PubTator to curate genes in PubMed abstracts. Database: J Biol Databases Curation 2012;2012:bas041.

[14] Li C, Liakata M, Rebholz-Schuhmann D. Biological network extraction from scientific literature: state of the art and challenges. Brief Bioinform 2014;15:856–77.

[15] Andronis C, et al. Literature mining, ontologies and information visualization for drug repurposing. Brief Bioinform 2011;12:357–68.

[16] Nováček V, Burns GAPC. SKIMMR: facilitating knowledge discovery in life sciences by machine-aided skim reading. PeerJ 2014;2:e483.

[17] Kilicoglu H, et al. Constructing a semantic predication gold standard from the biomedical literature. BMC Bioinformatics 2011;12:486.

[18] Wang H, et al. Finding complex biological relationships in recent PubMed articles using Bio-LDA. PLoS One 2011;6:e17243.

[19] Berman JJ. Pathology abbreviated: a long review of short terms. Arch Pathol Lab Med 2004;128(3):347–52.

[20] Ortutay C, Vihinen M. Immunome Knowledge Base (IKB): an integrated service for immunome research. BMC Immunol 2009;10(1):3.

[21] QIAGEN. Ingenuity pathway analysis. Available from: <http://www.ingenuity.com/>.

[22] Whirl-Carrillo M, et al. Pharmacogenomics knowledge for personalized medicine. Clin Pharmacol Ther 2012;92:414–17.

[23] Carbo A, et al. Predictive computational modeling of the mucosal immune responses during *Helicobacter pylori* infection. PLoS One 2013;8(9):e73365.

[24] Carbo A, et al. Systems modeling of molecular mechanisms controlling cytokine-driven CD4+ T cell differentiation and phenotype plasticity. PLoS Comput Biol 2013;9(4): e1003027.

[25] Carbo A, et al. Systems modeling of the role of interleukin-21 in the maintenance of effector CD4+ T cell responses during chronic *Helicobacter pylori* infection. MBio 2014;5(4): e01243–14

[26] Economou M, Pappas G. New global map of Crohn's disease: genetic, environmental, and socioeconomic correlations. Inflamm Bowel Dis 2008;14(5):709–20.

[27] Radivoyevitch T. Mass action models versus the Hill model: an analysis of tetrameric human thymidine kinase 1 positive cooperativity. Biol Direct 2009;4:49.

[28] Le DH, Kwon YK. A coherent feedforward loop design principle to sustain robustness of biological networks. Bioinformatics 2013;29(5):630–7.

[29] Mangan S, Alon U. Structure and function of the feed-forward loop network motif. Proc Natl Acad Sci USA 2003;100(21):11980–5.

[30] Barik D, et al. A model of yeast cell-cycle regulation based on multisite phosphorylation. Mol Syst Biol 2010;6:405.

[31] Qu Z, Weiss JN, MacLellan WR. Regulation of the mammalian cell cycle: a model of the G1-to-S transition. Am J Physiol Cell Physiol 2003;284(2):C349–64.

[32] Kapuy O, et al. Bistability by multiple phosphorylation of regulatory proteins. Prog Biophys Mol Biol 2009;100(1–3):47–56.

[33] Yang E, et al. Decay rates of human mRNAs: correlation with functional characteristics and sequence attributes. Genome Res 2003;13(8):1863–72.

[34] Hewitt M, et al. Ensuring confidence in predictions: a scheme to assess the scientific validity of in silico models. Adv Drug Deliv Rev 2015;86:101–11.

[35] Brown D, et al. Trauma *in silico*: individual-specific mathematical models and virtual clinical populations. Sci Transl Med 2015;7(285):285ra61.

[36] Sahle S, et al. A new strategy for assessing sensitivities in biochemical models. Philos Trans A Math Phys Eng Sci 2008;366(1880):3619–31.

[37] Kent E, Hoops S, Mendes P. Condor-COPASI: high-throughput computing for biochemical networks. BMC Syst Biol 2012;6(1):91.

[38] Carbo A, et al. Computational modeling of heterogeneity and function of CD4+ T cells. Front Cell Dev Biol 2014;2:31.

[39] Viladomiu M, et al. Modeling the role of peroxisome proliferator-activated receptor gamma and microRNA-146 in mucosal immune responses to *Clostridium difficile*. PLoS One 2012;7 (10):e47525.

[40] Kronsteiner B, et al. *Helicobacter pylori* infection in a pig model is dominated by Th1 and cytotoxic CD8 + T cell responses. Infect Immun 2013;81(10):3803–13.

[41] Bassaganya-Riera J, et al. *Helicobacter pylori* colonization ameliorates glucose homeostasis in mice through a PPAR gamma-dependent mechanism. PLoS One 2012;7(11):e50069.

[42] Lu P, et al. Computational modeling-based discovery of novel classes of anti-inflammatory drugs that target lanthionine synthetase C-like protein 2. PLoS One 2012;7(4):e34643.

[43] Philipson CW, Bassaganya-Riera J, Hontecillas R. Animal models of enteroaggregative *Escherichia coli* infection. Gut Microbes 2013;4(4):281–91.

[44] Higdon D, et al. Computer model calibration using high-dimensional output. J Am Stat Assoc 2008;103(482).

[45] Koehler JR, Owen AB. 9 Computer experiments. In: Ghosh S, Rao CR, editors. Handbook of Statistics 13: Design and Analysis of Experiments. North-Holland: Elsevier; 1996. p. 261–308. ISBN: 978-0-444-82061-7. http://www.sciencedirect.com/science/handbooks/01697161/13.

[46] Morris MD, Mitchell TJ. Exploratory designs for computational experiments. J Stat Plan Inference 1995;43(3):381–402.

[47] Lutz MW, et al. Experimental design for high-throughput screening. Drug Discov Today 1996;1(7):277–86.

[48] Smith DE, Mauro CA. Factor screening in computer simulation. Simulation 1982;38 (2):49–54.

[49] Borwein JM, Lewis AS. Convex analysis and nonlinear optimization: theory and examples, vol. 3. New York: Springer; 2010.

[50] Boyd S, Vandenberghe L. Convex optimization. New York, NY: Cambridge University Press; 2009.

[51] Craven MW, Shavlik JW. Using neural networks for data mining. Future Generation Comput Syst 1997;13(2):211–29.

[52] Lu H, Setiono R, Liu H. Effective data mining using neural networks. IEEE Trans Knowl Data Eng 1996;8(6):957–61.

[53] Dayhoff JE, DeLeo JM. Artificial neural networks. Cancer 2001;91(S8):1615–35.

[54] Ling H, Samarasinghe S, Kulasiri D. Novel recurrent neural network for modelling biological networks: oscillatory p53 interaction dynamics. Biosystems 2013;114(3):191–205.

[55] Snow PB, Smith DS, Catalona WJ. Artificial neural networks in the diagnosis and prognosis of prostate cancer: a pilot study. J Urol 1994;152(5 Pt 2):1923–6.

[56] Lek S, Guégan J-F. Artificial neural networks as a tool in ecological modelling, an introduction. Ecol Modell 1999;120(2):65–73.

[57] Brusic V, Rudy G, Harrison LC. Prediction of MHC binding peptides using artificial neural networks. Complex Syst: Mech Adaptation 1994;253–60.

[58] Lu P, Abedi V, Mei Y, Hontecillas R, Philipson C, Hoops S, et al. Supervised learning with artificial neural network in modeling of cell differentiation process. In: Tran QN, Arabnia H, editors. Emerging trends in computational biology, bioinformatics, and systems biology. 1st ed Burlington, Massachusetts: Morgan Kaufmann; 2015. p. 1–18.

[59] Lu P, et al. Supervised learning methods in modeling of CD4+ T cell heterogeneity. BioData Min 2015;8:27.

[60] Benedict KF, Lauffenburger DA. Insights into proteomic immune cell signaling and communication via data-driven modeling. Curr Top Microbiol Immunol 2013;363:201–33.

[61] Davison DB, et al. Whither computational biology. J Comput Biol 1994;1(1):1–2.

[62] Brown CT, et al. New computational approaches for analysis of cis-regulatory networks. Dev Biol 2002;246(1):86–102.

[63] Yuh CH, Bolouri H, Davidson EH. Genomic cis-regulatory logic: experimental and computational analysis of a sea urchin gene. Science 1998;279(5358):1896–902.

[64] Kitano H. Computational systems biology. Nature 2002;420(6912):206–10.

[65] Hucka M, et al. The systems biology markup language (SBML): a medium for representation and exchange of biochemical network models. Bioinformatics 2003;19(4):524–31.

[66] Hoops S, et al. COPASI—a complex pathway simulator. Bioinformatics 2006;22(24):3067–74.

[67] Mendes P, et al. Computational modeling of biochemical networks using COPASI. Methods Mol Biol 2009;500:17–59.

[68] Gillespie DT. A general method for numerically simulating the stochastic time evolution of coupled chemical reactions. J Comput Phys 1976;22(4):403–34.

[69] Gillespie DT. Exact stochastic simulation of coupled chemical reactions. J Phys Chem 1977;81(25):2340–61.

[70] Colby DA, Bergman RG, Ellman JA. Synthesis of dihydropyridines and pyridines from imines and alkynes via CH activation. J Am Chem Soc 2008;130(11):3645–51.

[71] Menolascina F, et al. Developing optimal input design strategies in cancer systems biology with applications to microfluidic device engineering. BMC Bioinformatics 2009;10(Suppl. 12):S4.

[72] Orton R, et al. Computational modelling of cancerous mutations in the EGFR/ERK signalling pathway. BMC Syst Biol 2009;3(1):100.

[73] Colvin RA, et al. Insights into Zn^{2+} homeostasis in neurons from experimental and modeling studies. Am J Physiol Cell Physiol 2008;294(3):C726–42.

[74] Nakano T, et al. A kinetic model of dopamine- and calcium-dependent striatal synaptic plasticity. PLoS Comput Biol 2010;6(2):e1000670.

[75] Ricagno S, et al. Human neuroserpin: structure and time-dependent inhibition. J Mol Biol 2009;388(1):109–21.

[76] Cimetiere N, Dossier-Berne F, De Laat J. Monochloramination of resorcinol: mechanism and kinetic modeling. Environ Sci Technol 2009;43(24):9380–5.

[77] Figueiredo AS, et al. Modelling and simulating interleukin-10 production and regulation by macrophages after stimulation with an immunomodulator of parasitic nematodes. FEBS J 2009;276(13):3454–69.

[78] Jordao L, et al. On the killing of mycobacteria by macrophages. Cell Microbiol 2007;10 (2):529–48.

[79] Curien G, et al. Understanding the regulation of aspartate metabolism using a model based on measured kinetic parameters. Mol Syst Biol 2009;5(1).

[80] Modre-Osprian R, et al. Dynamic simulations on the mitochondrial fatty acid beta-oxidation network. BMC Syst Biol 2009;3(1):2.

[81] Ma H, Boogerd FC, Goryanin I. Modelling nitrogen assimilation of *Escherichia coli* at low ammonium concentration. J Biotechnol 2009;144(3):175–83.

[82] Pingoud V, et al. On the divalent metal ion dependence of DNA cleavage by restriction endonucleases of the EcoRI family. J Mol Biol 2009;393(1):140–60.

[83] Blackmond DG. An examination of the role of autocatalytic cycles in the chemistry of proposed primordial reactions. Angewandte Chemie 2008;121(2):392–6.

[84] Iacus SM. Simulation and inference for stochastic differential equations: with R examples. New York: Springer; 2008. ISBN 978-0-387-75839-8.

[85] Chen KC, Wang TY, Tseng HH, Huang CY, Kao CY. A stochastic differential equation model for quantifying transcriptional regulatory network in *Saccharomyces cerevisiae*. Bioinformatics 2005;21(12):2883–90.

[86] Macarthur BD, Ma'ayan A, Lemischka IR. Systems biology of stem cell fate and cellular reprogramming. Nat Rev Mol Cell Biol 2009;10(10):672–81.

[87] MacArthur BD, Please CP, Oreffo RO. Stochasticity and the molecular mechanisms of induced pluripotency. PLoS One 2008;3(8):e3086.

[88] Manninen T, Linne ML, Ruohonen K. Developing Ito stochastic differential equation models for neuronal signal transduction pathways. Comput Biol Chem 2006;30(4):280–91.

[89] Saarinen A, Linne ML, Yli-Harja O. Stochastic differential equation model for cerebellar granule cell excitability. PLoS Comput Biol 2008;4(2):e1000004.

[90] Bisset KR, et al. High-performance interaction-based simulation of gut immunopathologies with ENteric immunity simulator (ENISI). 26th IEEE international parallel and distributed processing symposium, IPDPS 2012. Shanghai: IEEE Computer Society; 2012. Available from: http://dx.doi.org/10.1109/IPDPS.2012.15.

[91] Wendelsdorf K, et al. ENteric Immunity SImulator version 0.9: a tool for *in silico* study of gut immunopathologies. Blacksburg: NDSSL; 2011.

[92] Yongguo Mei RH, Zhang X, et al. ENISI Visual, an agent-based simulator for modeling gut immunity. IEEE international conference on bioinformatics and biomedicine (BIBM 2012). Philadelphia, PA; 2012.

[93] North M, et al. Complex adaptive systems modeling with Repast Simphony. Complex Adaptive Syst Model 2013;1(1):3.

[94] Yongguo M, et al. ENISI SDE: A New Web-Based Tool for Modeling Stochastic Processes. IEEE/ACM Trans. Comput. Biol. Bioinform. 2015;12(2):289–97.

[95] Mei Y, et al. Multiscale modeling of mucosal immune responses. BMC Bioinformatics 2015;16(Suppl. 12):S2.

[96] Barrett C, Bisset K, Eubank S, Feng X, Marathe M. EpiSimdemics: an efficient algorithm for simulating the spread of infectious disease over large realistic social networks. In: SuperComputing 08 INternational conference for high performance computing, networking, storage, and analysis. Austin, TX; 2008.

[97] Eubank S, et al. Modelling disease outbreaks in realistic urban social networks. Nature 2004;429(6988):180–4.

[98] Wendelsdorf K, et al. ENteric Immunity SImulator: a tool for *in silico* study of gastroenteric infections. IEEE Trans NanoBioScience 2012;11:273–88.

CHAPTER 3

Use of Computational Modeling in Immunological Research

Raquel Hontecillas[1], Josep Bassaganya-Riera[1], Casandra Philipson[2], Andrew Leber[1], Monica Viladomiu[1], Adria Carbo[2], Katherine Wendelsdorf[3], and Stefan Hoops[1]

[1]Nutritional Immunology and Molecular Medicine Laboratory, Virginia Bioinformatics Institute, Virginia Tech, Blacksburg, VA, USA [2]Biotherapeutics Inc., Blacksburg, VA, USA [3]Applied Advanced Genomics, QIAGEN, Redwood City, CA, USA

INTRODUCTION

Studying the mechanisms underlying immune responses has always been challenging due to the complexity of the immune system. The immune system can be broadly defined as an array of cells and organs whose main role is to distinguish self from nonself (pathogens) or altered self (cancer). This concept is several steps forward from the classical recognition of immunity as an organism's ability to defend itself from foreign invaders, that is, bacteria, viruses, or fungi. Immunologists have traditionally used mutually exclusive dichotomies to define and classify immune cells and functions. For instance CD4 + versus CD8 + T cells, or innate versus acquired immunity. However, advances in the past 15−20 years have torn down many of these conceptual divisions and uncovered a rather entangled system of cells, molecules, and functions. A very clear example is the initial Th1 versus Th2 classification of CD4 + T helper cells by Mossman in 1986 [1], which has evolved into the recognition that mature CD4 + T cells are intrinsically plastic and can adopt several functionalities depending on the context [2]. Even more recently, high-throughput technologies have allowed broad profiling of the changes occurring during immune responses at the organ, cell, protein, RNA, or gene levels. An early finding in this new era has been the recognition that nonimmune function-associated genes also play a significant role during the immune response and has open new areas of investigation, such as

Computational Immunology: Models and Tools. DOI: http://dx.doi.org/10.1016/B978-0-12-803697-6.00003-5

the metabolic control of inflammation and immune processes [3–6]. The biggest challenge of this new era is how to analyze, interpret, and extract new knowledge from this massive amount of data. Computational immunology can be envisioned as a logical continuation and adaptation to this new era, and a natural extension encompassing bioinformatics analysis. The great opportunity in front of us is the development of systems that will accelerate in an unprecedented manner new discoveries in basic immunological concepts as well as in the identification of targets for therapeutic applications.

COMPUTATIONAL AND MATHEMATICAL MODELING OF THE IMMUNE RESPONSE TO *HELICOBACTER PYLORI*

Helicobacter pylori is a Gram-negative, microaerophilic bacterium of the Epsilonproteobacteria that colonizes the stomach of nearly a half of the world's population. The presence of *H. pylori* in the stomach has been associated with various gastric diseases: gastritis, peptic ulcer disease, gastric adenocarcinoma, and gastric mucosa–associated lymphoma [7]. One of the most intriguing aspects of this human–bacteria interaction is that *H. pylori* colonizes the stomach chronically in spite of eliciting a detectable immunoinflammatory response. Its ability to conquer the stomach and survive in the gastric niche is tightly connected to avoiding the stomach low pH and the expression of various pathogenicity factors that enable adherence and penetration of the epithelial cell layer as well as immune evasion. In regards to the latter, the manipulation of innate and adaptive immune responses contributes to persistence and immunopathology in a way that is not fully understood. Moreover, though initially considered strictly a pathogen, there is growing evidence suggesting that the immune response to *H. pylori* has beneficial effects by protecting from inflammatory diseases like asthma, inflammatory bowel disease (IBD), esophageal cancer, or type-2 diabetes [8–10].

To facilitate a better understanding of the mechanisms underlying the interaction with the gastric environment at the systems levels, we constructed ordinary differential equation (ODE) model and agent-based model (ABM) depicting the immune response to *H. pylori*. As a starting point, we constructed an SBML network representing the major effector and regulatory cellular networks evoked during *H. pylori* infection [11] based on an extensive literature review. The model is comprised of four distinct anatomical compartments: the lumen, epithelium, gastric LP, and gastric lymph nodes (GLNs). The same network was used for ODE and ABM modeling approaches. In essence, the network is a representation of the connections between effector and regulatory cells in these compartments. As effector cells, we included M1 macrophages, Th1, Th17, and pro-inflammatory epithelial cells which secrete cytokines and chemokines that (i) recruit immune cells, (ii) promote activation and differentiation to inflammatory phenotypes, and (iii) secrete effector molecules that eliminate bacteria and may cause tissue damage. Regulatory cells such as M2 macrophages, tolerogenic dendritic cells (DCs), and Treg cells act antagonistically to their inflammatory/effector counterparts through various contact- and cytokine-dependent mechanisms [12–14]. All populations were further separated by location in the described compartments (GLN, gastric LP, epithelium, and lumen).

Our computational model represents the migration of *H. pylori* from the mucus layer of the gastric lumen toward the epithelium and the invasion of the LP. However, upon contact of the bacterium with a healthy epithelial cell, represented as E, bacterial infection is initiated and this epithelial cell starts secreting inflammatory mediators, represented as E_damaged in the network model, thus triggering an inflammatory response affecting mainly effector cells. Tolerogenic bacteria (TolB) are also represented, highlighting how commensalism helps to maintain a regulatory phenotype at the gut mucosa (Figure 3.1).

Once the network was completed, the CellDesigner-based SBML model was imported into COPASI, parametrized and calibrated by assigning specific values to each of the model species obtained from the literature or generated in house. At this point, it could be used for conducting *in silico* experiments. One topic of active research in the immune response to *H. pylori* has been the role of macrophages in pathology and persistence [15,16]. The model was used to generate an *in silico* knockout system in which PPARγ, a transcription factor that opposes pathways that upregulate pro-inflammatory genes, was deleted in myeloid cells represented in the model. An interesting outcome of the *in silico* experiment was that the loss of PPARγ leads to lower levels of colonization. We then run an experiment comparing WT and PPARγ$^{fl/fl}$; Lys-M^{Cre} mice (myeloid PPARγ KO mouse) and were able to validate this prediction of the model. With this modeling exercise

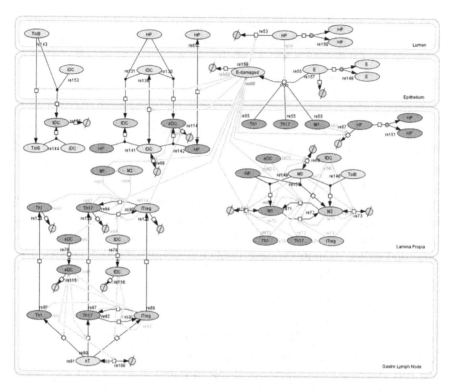

Figure 3.1 **Network model of the mucosal immune responses during** Helicobacter **pylori** *infection. Systems Biology Markup Language (SBML)-compliant network of the interactions between H. pylori and cells participating in the innate and adaptive immune response such as macrophages (M1 and M2), dendritic cells (tDC and eDC), epithelial cells (E), and CD4+ T cell subsets (Th1, Th17, iTreg) in the gastric lumen, the epithelium, lamina propria (LP), and the gastric lymph nodes (GLNs).*

we have been able to generate new hypothesis, although the exact cellular or molecular mechanisms were unknown. An efficient way to approach follow-up experiments is to perform a sensitivity analysis in order to rank immunological parameters of the model by their relevance in the system's dynamics and outcome. The result has been the identification of epithelial cells and macrophages as the key cells of the system driving the outcome of the interaction [17]. The great majority of *H. pylori* in the gastric mucosa is found free-floating in the mucus layer and associated with the apical side of epithelial cells [18,19]. Thus, the model recapitulates this principle and the sensitivity analysis indicates that the epithelium is the compartment that receives the major impact of the infection. An interesting and less intuitive finding of the model is the relationship between epithelium and macrophages. The model also predicted that applying different values of epithelial cell activation, *H. pylori* leads to a sequential accumulation of macrophage precursors (M0) between days 0 and 14/21 postinfection. This first wave is followed by a subset of M2 with regulatory/suppressor role, which peaks between days 21 and 35 postinfection. Interestingly, we have recently identified a subset of macrophages with regulatory suppressor phenotype that facilitates *H. pylori* colonization leading to high stomach burden.

In summary, computational modeling has allowed us to perform cost-efficient *in silico* experiments that, although have not provided detailed mechanistic insights in the interaction of *H. pylori* with the gastric mucosa, have guided experimentalists by narrowing down the elements of the system that have the greatest influence in the outcome of the infection.

INFLAMMATORY BOWEL DISEASE

IBD is a chronic autoimmune disease comprised of Crohn's disease and ulcerative colitis that afflicts approximately 1.4 million people in the United States and more than 4 million people worldwide. IBD onset results as a consequence of several improperly balanced processes such as misguided cross talk between the host and gut commensal microbiota. Genetic susceptibility and dysregulated immune responses can result in an imbalance between effector and regulatory pathways in the gut also contributing to the initiation of IBD.

We generated an ODE and ABM biological system to mathematically model cross talk between inflammatory and regulatory pathways in the gut during IBD [20]. As outlined above, the ODE model and ABM utilized the same network and yielded similar immunological findings. Within the systems, commensal bacteria recognized as residential, guide the development of regulatory immune cells and assist in a healthy homeostatic balance. Regulatory DCs, macrophages (M2), and T cells (Treg) contribute tolerogenic responses to beneficial microbes and negatively regulate inflammation. In contrast, commensal bacteria that are recognized as pathogenic by the host trigger inflammatory pathways. More specifically, when antigen-presenting cells (i.e., macrophages or DCs) come into contact with harmful commensals, these phagocytes engulf the bacteria and differentiate into activated effector phenotypes: M1 and De. Moreover, upon activation these effector cell types will secrete cytokines, which further exacerbate pro-inflammatory responses. Through antigen presentation and chemical signaling, effector CD4 Th1 and Th17 phenotypes act synergistically with M1 and De in another positive feedback loop to recruit additional infiltrating monocytes and potentiate lesion formation *in silico* in the colonic tissue (Figure 3.2).

We performed a series of *in silico* experiments using the IBD model and predicted that macrophage phenotypes were unfavorably plastic, especially under chronic inflammatory setting triggered by gut microflora, and could be positively manipulated using PPARγ as an immune modulator. Another key computational prediction stemming from the original insight highlighted a central role of M1 in robust hyperactivation of inflammation through an unforeseen feedback loop governing T-cell responses. Concisely, T-cell-targeted mechanisms were ineffective in rescuing IBD in our computational model. On the other hand, the M1 phenotype represented a highly efficacious target for

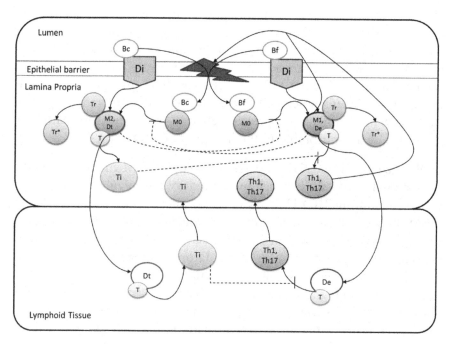

*Figure 3.2 **Network model of the mucosal immune responses during inflammatory bowel disease.** Biological cross talk between inflammatory and regulatory signaling pathways in the colon is represented at the lumen, epithelial barrier, lamina propria, and lymph node compartments. Solid lines indicate positive regulation whereas dashed lines represent negative signaling. Beneficial (Bc) and harmful (Bf) commensal bacteria initiate signaling to dendritic cells (De, Dt) and macrophages (M0, M1, M2) ultimately orchestrating T-cell phenotypes.*

immune-mediated therapy. Two scenarios were tested through *in silico* trials to evaluate the therapeutic value of targeting macrophage processes as a means to treat autoimmunity associated with IBD. First, monocyte recruitment was reduced, however this caused more sustained severity with respect to damaged epithelium and activating cytokine levels. Our second mechanism for investigation was to reduce the ability for antigen-presenting cells to stimulate memory in activated CD4+ T-cell populations. Removing this signaling mechanism entirely also resulted in loss of epithelial integrity, however minimizing stimulation of T cells by effector antigen-presenting cells only (M1, De) promoted almost complete restoration of immune and epithelial cells.

In summary, our overall objective was to characterize nonintuitive interactions between contrasting effector and regulatory processes that ultimately resulted in identifying the potential for macrophages to be more potent targets for therapy rather than T cells. Subsequent studies in our laboratory demonstrated that one beneficial role of probiotic bacteria is to produce PPAR ligands that suppress colitis in a macrophage-dependent manner, validating the model predictions presented above [21]. Taken together, this model represents an integration of experimental data and mathematical modeling to generate new knowledge for characterizing host immunity.

ODE MODEL OF CD4+ T-CELL DIFFERENTIATION

In addition to the described tissue-level models, which simulate interaction of cells embedded in tissues, we have also constructed single-cell models that represent molecular events leading to a specific functional phenotype as outcome. A good example of such model is the differentiation of CD4+ T cells based on external cytokine environment and subsequent changes in cytoplasmic molecular signaling. CD4+ T helper cells are a population of lymphocytes that contribute to the initiation, maintenance, and cessation of immune responses. The CD4+ T-cell family is divided into numerous subsets with varying degrees of effector and regulatory functionalities. Noticeable changes in the proportions of these subsets occur in response to bacterial and viral agents, which are mainly transmitted by cytokines secreted by epithelial or mononuclear phagocytes coming in contact with microbial determinants. In addition, the dysregulation of a balanced CD4+ T-cell composition can be associated with the development of autoimmune and inflammatory disease.

The activation and differentiation of CD4+ T cells can occur through direct interactions with antigen-presenting cells and sensing of the extracellular cytokine milieu. However, the commitment to one phenotype is not terminal. Instead, differentiated CD4+ T cells remain plastic and continue to shift their behavior according to interactions with the local environment.

A massively interacting network of molecular events is responsible for driving the activation of transcription factors in response to cytokine signaling, which ultimately determine the secretory behavior of a differentiated CD4+ T cell (Figure 3.3). The creation of a computational model describing this system has greatly enhanced the understanding of the network and ability to elucidate the roles of molecules within the system. The model details the differentiation into one of four phenotypes: T helper 1 (Th1), T helper 2 (Th2), T helper 17 (Th17), and regulatory (iTreg). In general, the network proceeds according to the following hierarchy of events. A pool of extracellular cytokines exists and can be sensed through a binding to receptors located on the cell surface. The resultant complex activates or inhibits

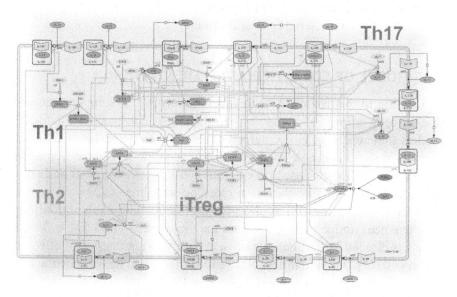

Figure 3.3 **Network model of CD4+ T-cell differentiation.** *SBML-compliant network illustrating the signaling and transcriptional pathways from the binding of extracellular cytokines to the activation of transcription factors define the differentiation of a CD4+ T cell. Arrows mark transitions, green lines mark activation, and red lines mark inhibitions. The model describes differentiation into Th1, Th2, Th17, and iTreg phenotypes. (For interpretation of the references to color in this figure legend, the reader is referred to the web version of this book.)*

signal-transducing proteins, such as the STAT family of proteins. In an activated state, the signal-transducing proteins in turn activate canonical transcription factors (T-bet, GATA-3, FoxP3, and RORγT) for each of the cell subset. The activation of transcription factors controls the production of cytokines, which are then secreted into the extracellular environment. The model continues in an uninterrupted cycle allowing the system to progress toward a steady state.

Following calibration, the initial model was used to investigate the ability of PPARγ to control the balance between regulatory and effector subsets [22]. With an *in silico* knockout of PPARγ, simulations displayed that an increased prevalence of Th17 cells would exist, suggesting a role for PPARγ in determining the balance between Th17 and iTreg. Our cell-based model is generic in the sense that it represents CD4+ T-cell differentiation out of any particular context. However, when the model was then recalibrated using data specific for an *H. pylori* challenge we could perform simulations on CD4+ T-cell differentiation during bacterial infection [23]. Experimentation with the recalibrated model aimed to explore the effect of IL-21, which is important not only in the control of *H. pylori* but also in the establishment of chronic inflammation, on the CD4+ T-cell response. Sensitivity analysis of the model displayed that the presence of IL-21 would have a largest positive effect on the production of IL-17, the activation of RORγT, and the phosphorylation of STAT3; three events that are associated with a Th17 population. Smaller positive effects were displayed with the Th1-associated T-bet and IFNγ, while negative effects were predicted on the iTreg-associated FoxP3 and IL-10. In addition, a simulated knockout of IL-21 projected large shifts in the activation of these molecules, which was later confirmed with good agreement by a small *in vivo* study.

T FOLLICULAR HELPER CELL DIFFERENTIATION

Maintaining a balance between effector and regulatory responses is important in the prevention of immune-mediated disease development and reactiveness to the native microbiota [24,25]. A critical controller of this balance may be a population of CD4+ T cells, known as T follicular helper (Tfh) cells due to their ability to localize to and interact with cells within germinal follicles [26]. Through the canonical transcription factor Bcl-6, Tfh cells are able to produce a number of pro-inflammatory cytokines, such as IL-21, a potent mediator of gastric inflammation in response *H. pylori* colonization [23,27]. However, the generation and stability of the Tfh population is regulated by a separate CD4+ T-cell subset, T follicular regulatory (Tfr) cells [28].

The presence of two antagonistic cell types could suggest the presence of bistability within the system of interactions. Therefore, a computational model to explore the events surrounding the differentiation of these two cell types was developed. Initially, a small model containing seven nodes was created. This model described the differentiation of Tfh and Tfr subsets from respective precursor cells, naïve CD4+ T and Treg cells. These populations were controlled by the expression and interactions between transcription regulators Bcl-6 and Blimp-1 as well as the chemokine receptor CXCR5. After local stability analysis and simulations, the model was expanded (Figure 3.4)

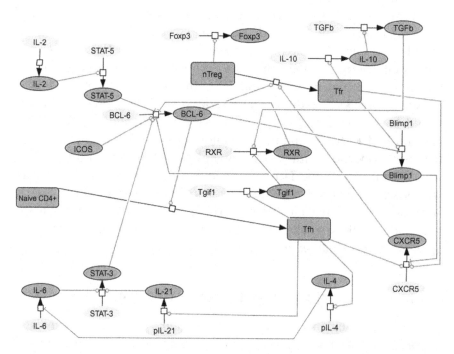

*Figure 3.4 **Network model of T follicular helper cell differentiation.** The differentiation of CD4+ T follicular helper (Tfh) and T follicular regulatory (Tfr) cells is controlled by the expression of transcription factors Bcl-6 and Blimp1. The cells also contribute to the production of cytokines (IL-4, IL-6, IL-10, IL-21) and other proteins (Foxp3, CXCR5, Tgif1, RXR). Black arrows mark transitions, green connections mark activation, and red connections mark inhibition. The interactions within the network create bistable dynamics between a high and a low Tfh state. (For interpretation of the references to color in this figure legend, the reader is referred to the web version of this book.)*

while keeping the core interactions intact. The model expanded to include cytokine signaling pathways, involving cytokines such as IL-21, IL-6, IL-4, and IL-10, to drive the activation of Bcl-6 within the model. For example, the production of IL-21 by Tfh cells activates STAT-3 that in turn activates Bcl-6.

After calibration with a combination of *in vitro* and *in vivo* data, the small model displayed that a bistable range existed between two steady states. These two steady states showed large differences between the two Tfh populations: one in which the Tfh population was nearly zero and one in which the Tfh population was stably and chronically elevated. The expansion of the network allowed for the exploration of new pathways that would exacerbate or resolve the chronically elevated Tfh population. After assessing a number of potential additions through sensitivity analysis, a pathway involving Tgif1 was identified as having the highest potential impact. The increased expression of Tgif1 would inhibit the retinoid X receptor (RXR)-mediated inhibition of Bcl-6, creating a mechanism in which Tfh cells are able to maintain Bcl-6 activation and continual differentiation into the Tfh phenotype. After simulations, small changes in the parameters controlling Tgif1 activation were found to have a switch capability between the high and low steady states. In contrast, an impulse of RXR activation was found to return the chronically elevated Tfh population to healthy levels.

In summary, the creation of a network describing Tfh cell differentiation allowed for the observation of bistability within the network. Further expansion and analysis created opportunities to identify novel controllers of the commitment to a high or low Tfh steady state. This identification of new contributors to fate determination could lead to the development of potential treatments for chronic inflammation and alternatives to eradication of commensal species.

CONCLUDING REMARKS

In this chapter, we present examples of how computational modeling can be incorporated into immunological research. The models have been used to perform experiments testing new hypotheses *in silico* and to perform sensitivity analysis to guide *in vivo* experimentation. Technical details on how models were constructed are provided in

Chapters 5 and 6 dealing with ODE and ABM, respectively. These models provide an ideal framework to integrate diverse data types (i.e., flow cytometry, gene expression, pathology) that otherwise would have been presented as independent datasets. The integration of procedural knowledge and data across scales constitutes the basis for multiscale modeling that will be discussed in Chapter 8.

ACKNOWLEDGMENTS

This work was supported in part by National Institute of Allergy and Infectious Diseases Contract No. HHSN272201000056C to JBR and funds from the Nutritional Immunology and Molecular Medicine Laboratory (www.nimml.org).

REFERENCES

[1] Mosmann TR, Cherwinski H, Bond MW, Giedlin MA, Coffman RL. Two types of murine helper T cell clone. I. Definition according to profiles of lymphokine activities and secreted proteins. J Immunol 1986;136(7):2348–57.

[2] Geginat J, Paroni M, Maglie S, Alfen JS, Kastirr I, Gruarin P, et al. Plasticity of human CD4 T cell subsets. Front Immunol 2014;5:630.

[3] Ramsay G, Cantrell D. Environmental and metabolic sensors that control T cell biology. Front Immunol 2015;6:99.

[4] Pallett LJ, Gill US, Quaglia A, Sinclair LV, Jover-Cobos M, Schurich A, et al. Metabolic regulation of hepatitis B immunopathology by myeloid-derived suppressor cells. Nat Med 2015;21(6):591–600.

[5] Jin C, Henao-Mejia J, Flavell RA. Innate immune receptors: key regulators of metabolic disease progression. Cell Metab 2013;17(6):873–82.

[6] Granger A, Emambokus N. Focus on immunometabolism. Cell Metab 2013;17(6):807.

[7] Atherton JC, Blaser MJ. Coadaptation of *Helicobacter pylori* and humans: ancient history, modern implications. J Clin Invest 2009;119(9):2475–87.

[8] Pacifico L, Anania C, Osborn JF, Ferraro F, Chiesa C. Consequences of *Helicobacter pylori* infection in children. World J Gastroenterol 2010;16(41):5181–94.

[9] Bassaganya-Riera J, Dominguez-Bello MG, Kronsteiner B, Carbo A, Lu P, Viladomiu M, et al. *Helicobacter pylori* colonization ameliorates glucose homeostasis in mice through a PPAR gamma-dependent mechanism. PLoS One 2012;7(11):e50069.

[10] Arnold IC, Dehzad N, Reuter S, Martin H, Becher B, Taube C, et al. *Helicobacter pylori* infection prevents allergic asthma in mouse models through the induction of regulatory T cells. J Clin Invest 2011;121(8):3088–93.

[11] Funahashi A, Tanimura N, Morohashi M, Kitano H. CellDesigner: a process diagram editor for gene-regulatory and biochemical networks. BIOSILICO 2003;1:159–62.

[12] Iwasaki A. Mucosal dendritic cells. Annu Rev Immunol 2007;25:381–418.

[13] Ng SC, Kamm MA, Stagg AJ, Knight SC. Intestinal dendritic cells: their role in bacterial recognition, lymphocyte homing, and intestinal inflammation. Inflamm Bowel Dis 2010;16 (10):1787–807.

[14] Littman DR, Rudensky AY. Th17 and regulatory T cells in mediating and restraining inflammation. Cell 2010;140(6):845–58.

[15] Gobert AP, Verriere T, Asim M, Barry DP, Piazuelo MB, de Sablet T, et al. Heme oxygenase-1 dysregulates macrophage polarization and the immune response to *Helicobacter pylori*. J Immunol 2014;193(6):3013–22.

[16] Schumacher MA, Donnelly JM, Engevik AC, Xiao C, Yang L, Kenny S, et al. Gastric Sonic Hedgehog acts as a macrophage chemoattractant during the immune response to *Helicobacter pylori*. Gastroenterology 2012;142(5).

[17] Alam M, et al. Sensitivity Analysis of an ENteric Immunity SImulator (ENISI)-Based Model of Immune Responses to Helicobacter pylori Infection. PLoS One 2015;10(9): e0136139.

[18] Kronsteiner B, Bassaganya-Riera J, Philipson N, Hontecillas R. Novel insights on the role of CD8 + T cells and cytotoxic responses during *Helicobacter pylori* infection. Gut Microbes 2014;5(3).

[19] Sigal M, Rothenberg ME, Logan CY, Lee JY, Honaker RW, Cooper RL, et al. Helicobacter pylori Activates and Expands Lgr5(+) Stem Cells Through Direct Colonization of the Gastric Glands. Gastroenterology 2015;148:1392–404, e21.

[20] Wendelsdorf K, Bassaganya-Riera J, Hontecillas R, Eubank S. Model of colonic inflammation: immune modulatory mechanisms in inflammatory bowel disease. J Theor Biol 2010;264(4):1225–39.

[21] Bassaganya-Riera J, Viladomiu M, Pedragosa M, De Simone C, Carbo A, Shaykhutdinov R, et al. Probiotic bacteria produce conjugated linoleic acid locally in the gut that targets macrophage PPAR gamma to suppress colitis. PLoS One 2012;7(2):e31238.

[22] Carbo A, Hontecillas R, Kronsteiner B, Viladomiu M, Pedragosa M, Lu P, et al. Systems modeling of molecular mechanisms controlling cytokine-driven CD4+ T cell differentiation and phenotype plasticity. PLoS Comput Biol 2013;9(4):e1003027.

[23] Carbo A, Olivares-Villagomez D, Hontecillas R, Bassaganya-Riera J, Chaturvedi R, Piazuelo MB, et al. Systems modeling of the role of interleukin-21 in the maintenance of effector CD4+ T cell responses during chronic *Helicobacter pylori* infection. MBio 2014;5 (4): e01243-14.

[24] Belkaid Y, Rouse BT. Natural regulatory T cells in infectious disease. Nat Immunol 2005;6 (4):353–60.

[25] Zhou L, Chong MM, Littman DR. Plasticity of CD4+ T cell lineage differentiation. Immunity 2009;30(5):646–55.

[26] King C, Tangye SG, Mackay CR. T follicular helper (TFH) cells in normal and dysregulated immune responses. Annu Rev Immunol 2008;26:741–66.

[27] Nurieva R, Yang XO, Martinez G, Zhang Y, Panopoulos AD, Ma L, et al. Essential autocrine regulation by IL-21 in the generation of inflammatory T cells. Nature 2007;448 (7152):480–3.

[28] Linterman MA, Pierson W, Lee SK, Kallies A, Kawamoto S, Rayner TF, et al. Foxp3+ follicular regulatory T cells control the germinal center response. Nat Med 2011;17 (8):975–82.

CHAPTER 4

Immunoinformatics Cyberinfrastructure for Modeling and Analytics

Stefan Hoops[1], Bruno W. Sobral[2], Pawel Michalak[1], Vida Abedi[1], Barbara Kronsteiner[1], Raquel Hontecillas[1], Monica Viladomiu[1], and Josep Bassaganya-Riera[1]

[1]Nutritional Immunology and Molecular Medicine Laboratory, Virginia Bioinformatics Institute, Virginia Tech, Blacksburg, VA, USA [2]One Health Institute, Colorado State University, Fort Collins, CO, USA

INTRODUCTION

The bioinformatics infrastructure plays an important role in the systems approach to immunology research. Informatics infrastructure enables the research process from literature search, experimentation, model creation, calibration, analysis, and sharing. For enhanced community effectiveness it is crucial that all results are also made publicly available in repositories like Immport, GEO, or Biomodels.net. The Modeling Immunity to Enteric Pathogens (MIEP) has developed and is continuously improving a comprehensive web-based experimental environment that provides support and infrastructure to computational and experimental research.

The inner circle of Figure 4.1 presents the process of research from literature search, model development, *in silico* experiments, to wet-lab experiments, data processing, visualization, and publications. The outer circle shows the supporting bioinformatics technologies, including databases, data management, laboratory information management, data processing, data sharing, and Web portal.

The management and implementation of the infrastructure is driven from the user view. This means that it is of utmost importance to identify the stakeholders that will use the resource. After identifying the stakeholder, we define the high-level services that need to be provided to support the research process as depicted in Figure 4.1. These high-level services rely on low-level services such as security management

Computational Immunology: Models and Tools. DOI: http://dx.doi.org/10.1016/B978-0-12-803697-6.00004-7

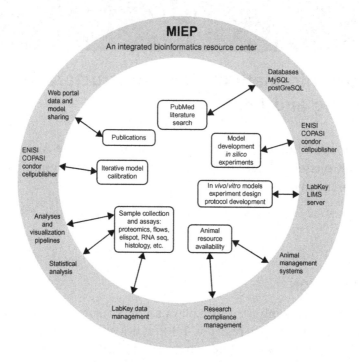

Figure 4.1 Research process supported by the Bioinformatics infrastructure.

and databases as well as access to workflows and internal and external knowledge repositories. The foundation of the bioinformatics infrastructure is provided by the hardware layer which is formed by networking, computing and storage components (Figure 4.2).

WEB PORTAL

The MIEP Web Portal (www.modelingimmunity.org) is the first-line tool for dissemination of research results such as publications, experimental results, and models. Additionally it functions as the central access point to all services provided by the bioinformatics team. These services are either available publicly or through the Intranet, which only accessible to team members and collaborators (Figure 4.3).

MIEP uses CellPublisher [1] to provide enriched visualization of the identified host tolerance networks and pathways (Figure 4.4). CellPublisher allows us to connect arbitrary meta-information to edges and nodes of the network.

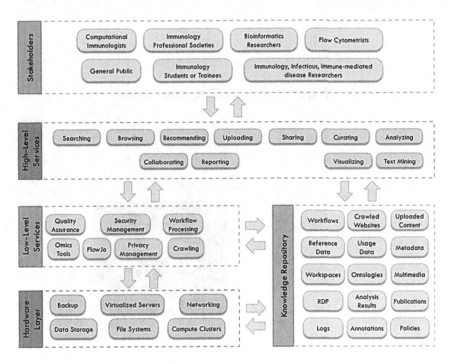

Figure 4.2 High-level architectural concept of the immunoinformatics infrastructure.

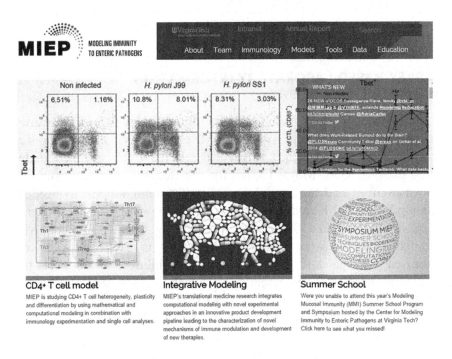

Figure 4.3 The MIEP Web portal which functions as the main dissemination and access point.

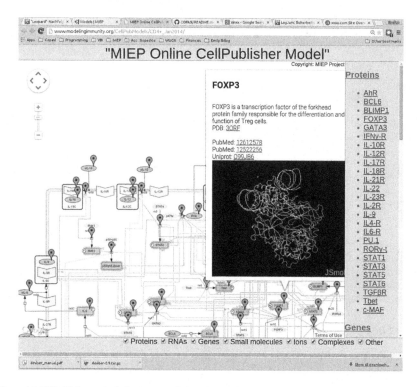

Figure 4.4 CellPublisher network showing a pathway of CD4+ T cells and the protein FOXP3 with references to publications in PubMed and the Uniprot entry.

LABKEY-BASED LABORATORY INFORMATION MANAGEMENT SYSTEM

A major component of the informatics infrastructure is the Laboratory Information Management System (LIMS), which uses the open-source software from LabKey [2]. LabKey was selected after a detailed analysis of existing tools. Major factors for our decision were the extensive documentation and the availability of professional support as needed. After piloting LabKey during the second year we moved it into production over the last 6 months. We recently updated our LabKey installation to the latest release and moved it to new hardware with increased storage and computational capabilities to support the increasing needs of our researchers, which include studies utilizing RNA-Seq, flow cytometry, ELISA, ELISPOT, microbiome, RT-PCR data. All ongoing studies are now managed in LabKey. The starting page for the EAEC-PO1 study as well a list of others on the left can be seen below (Figures 4.5 and 4.6).

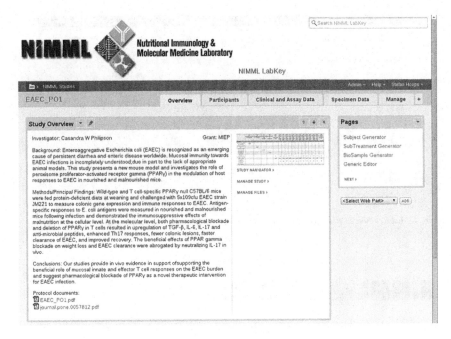

Figure 4.5 LabKey Interface. Home page of the EAEC_PO1 study.

	All Timepoints	Day -1	Day 0	Day 2	Day 6	Day 13	Day 20	Day 28	Day 35	Day 41	Day 48	Day 51	Day 55	Day 59
Subjects?	35		35											
Subject Treatments?	69		35	34										
Biological Samples?	301	35			34	34	34	34	34	34	34	9	9	10
Biological Sample Treatments?	28											9	9	10
Subject Diets?	0													

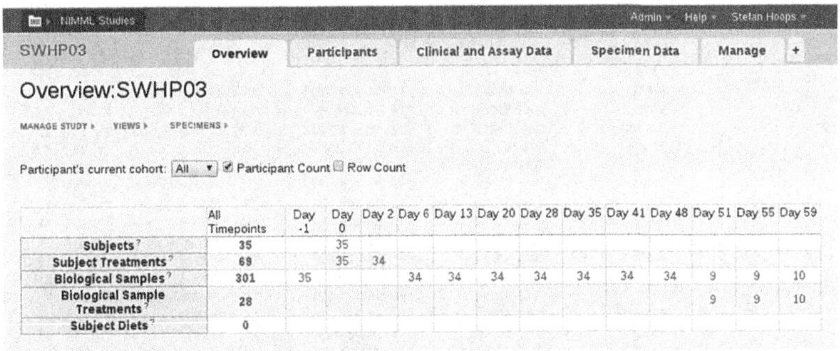

Figure 4.6 LabKey Study Navigator. The navigator provides easy access to subject and samples collected during a study.

Certain aspects of the laboratory work are common for all studies such as the list of available reagents or protocols and standard operating procedures (SOPs). SOPs are crucial to enable data integration and comparisons. We support this by establishing central tables with interface for the management of these components (Figure 4.7).

A majority of the subjects studied at MIEP are mice. It is therefore important for the experimenter to be able to select their study

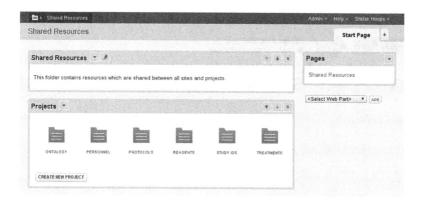

Figure 4.7 LabKey Shared Resources. Overview of the resources shared by all studies resources.

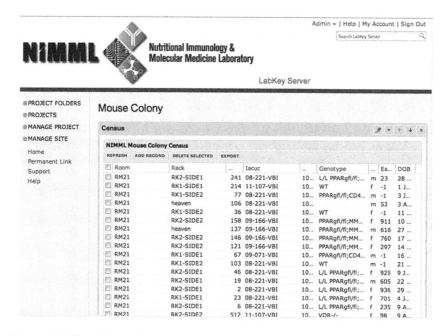

Figure 4.8 LabKey—Mouse Colony Integration. A list of currently available mice shown in the LabKey-based LIMS.

subjects from the mouse colony database (MouseDB). We have begun the integration by providing a list of mice available in the mouse colony for use in a study. In the future, the selected mice will be automatically inserted as subjects into the study in LIMS and marked in the MouseDB as used so that they cannot be selected again (Figure 4.8).

PUBLIC REPOSITORIES: IMMPORT

Our LIMS is designed in such a way that all required data for ImmPort submission is captured in real time, that is, the experimenter provides all relevant information when recording experimental steps and results. We implemented a controlled vocabulary, which is easily mapped to the ImmPort data. We would have preferred to use existing ontologies as they are provided by the MIRIAM registry. However, the mandate to map these rich and flexible annotations to limited Immport vocabulary was not feasible. To enhance the usability the user is provided with drop-down boxes wherever the input of controlled vocabulary data is required.

We have implemented PHP-based export tool (2ImmPort), which converts study data collected in LabKey to the ImmPort compliant tab separated file format and packages it in a zip file ready for ImmPort submission. We used the PHP tool 2ImmPort to generate submission packages for 20 studies (see Appendix) conducted over the last 5 years by the MIEP team which is more than 1/3 of the studies uploaded by the four centers participating in the NIAID funded effort Modeling Immunity for Biodefense (MIB).

GLOBAL GENE EXPRESSION ANALYSIS

Galaxy is an open, web-based platform to perform accessible, reproducible, and transparent NGS analyses, providing all the necessary tools to create and execute a complete RNA-Seq analysis pipeline. Users without programming experience can easily specify parameters and run tools and workflows. As part of the MIEP program, we have developed an automated RNA-Seq pipeline supported by a 96-core (Intel) cluster (Shadowfax), 64-bit, with 386 GB memory, and 60 TB of shared Panasas PAS7 disk space already assembled at Virginia Bioinformatics Institute. From the Galaxy page of MIEP website, internal users can access the new integrated tool. We have improved the upload performance of Galaxy for large data files (3 Gb RNA-Seq data) to allow researchers to analyze next-generation sequencing (NGS) results (Figure 4.9).

HIGH-PERFORMANCE COMPUTING ENVIRONMENT

HPC for Condor-COPASI. The model analysis, especially the parameter estimation, is a computing intensive process exceeding the

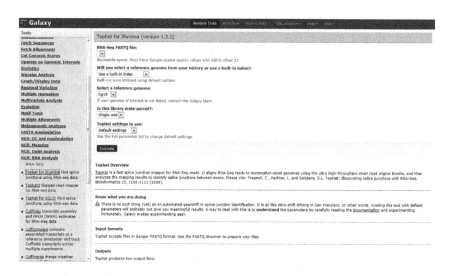

Figure 4.9 Galaxy RNA-seq analysis.

capabilities of the local computational infrastructure of many of the intended researchers. The general approach is to submit these computing extensive tasks to a high-performance computer or cluster. This approach commonly requires the researcher to interact with a command line based job submission system and manually transfer files and analyze results. To support our researchers we installed the open-source software Condor-COPASI, which provides an intuitive web interface for the submission of COPASI-based analysis jobs (Figure 4.4).

In the case of parameter estimation, Condor-COPASI allows the user to schedule repeats of jobs to provide statistics. The users only need to provide their COPASI file and the experimental data. Condor-COPASI automatically analyzes the result and returns the best fit. The user additionally provided with option to download a COPASI model representing this solution.

The MIEP team has successfully installed Condor-COPASI in VBI high-performance cluster Shadowfax. Condor-COPASI is configured in such a way that its users have priority access to the MIEP financed section but are not limited to it (Figure 4.10).

HPC INFRASTRUCTURE FOR ENISI MSM MODELING

The high-performance *in silico* experimentation is performed using HPC configured to run on Shadowfax (HPC cluster). This

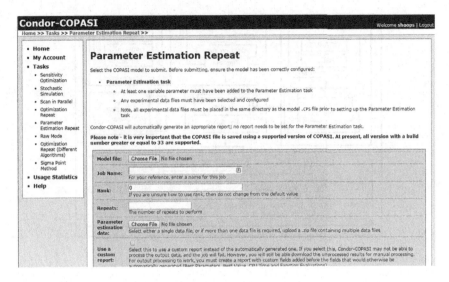

Figure 4.10 Condor-COPASI job submission interface for the parameter estimation repeat.

experimentation will test the scalability of large systems. The HPC cluster used consists of 170 dual-socket nodes, 2 quad-socket large memory nodes, and 8 special purpose FPGA (Field Programmable Gate Array) nodes. The system also includes two large memory nodes with 40 cores and 1 TB of memory each. There are also eight nodes with FPGA that provide accelerated genomics processing. We used Shadowfax to simulate 10^9 agents using only 100 cores. ENISI MSM has therefore the potential to scale to larger systems very efficiently. Further optimization is currently in progress to further enhance the capabilities of the system and use it for modeling more complex immune-mediated processes.

CYBERINFRASTRUCTURE FOR NETWORK SCIENCE

Networks are an effective abstraction for representing real systems. Consequently, network science is increasingly used in academia and industry to solve problems in many fields. Computations that determine structure properties and dynamical behaviors of networks are useful because they give insights into the characteristics of real systems. CINET [3,4], a CyberInfrastructure for NETwork science, is a web-based tool for analyzing networks that represent interactions in large-scale complex systems. It provides a large set of networks and

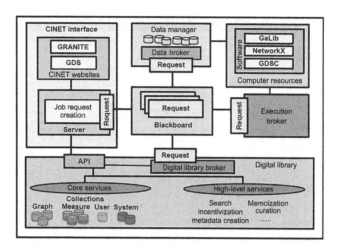

Figure 4.11 High-level overview of CINET system components and interactions.

algorithms to analyze them. Users can also add their own networks to be analyzed by the provided algorithms. This web-based interface has been designed to simplify analysis of complex networks for users who are not necessarily computer scientists (Figure 4.11).

PATHOSYSTEMS RESOURCE INTEGRATION CENTER

The Pathosystems Resource Integration Center (PATRIC) [5] (Figure 4.12) is the all-bacterial Bioinformatics Resource Center (BRC) (http://pathogenportal.org). A joint effort by two of the original National Institute of Allergy and Infectious Diseases funded BRCs, PATRIC provides researchers with an online resource that stores and integrates a variety of data types (e.g., genomics, transcriptomics, protein–protein interactions (PPIs), three-dimensional protein structures, and sequence typing data) and associated metadata. Data types are summarized for individual genomes and across taxonomic levels. All genomes in PATRIC, in July 2015 more than 30,000, have been consistently annotated using RAST, the Rapid Annotations using Subsystems Technology. Summaries of different data types are also provided for individual genes, where comparisons of different annotations are available, and also include available transcriptomic data. PATRIC provides a variety of ways for researchers to find data of interest and a

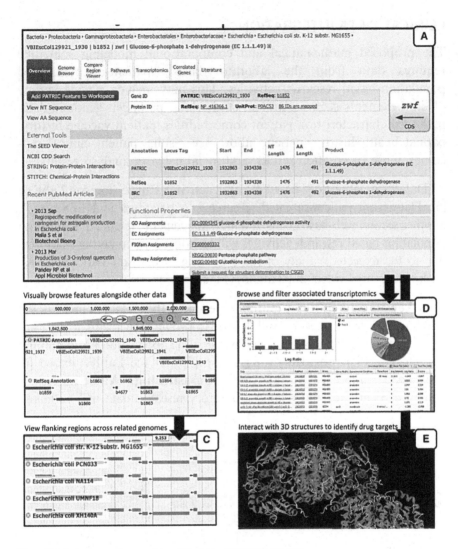

Figure 4.12 Pathosystems Resource Integration Center (PATRIC) use case.

private workspace where they can store both genomic and gene associations, and their own private data. Both private and public data can be analyzed together using a suite of tools to perform comparative genomic or transcriptomic analysis (as an upload, software as a service functionality designed for informatics-naïve users). PATRIC also includes integrated information related to disease and PPIs. All the data and integrated analysis and visualization tools are freely available.

CLINICAL DATA INTEGRATION

The proposed mathematical and computational modeling sometime requires data from the laboratory-based, patient-oriented, and population-based research activities. This may include a wide variety of data elements such as: animal study data, pathogen genomic data, pathogen characteristics, patient comorbidities, patient vaccine history, patient health history, patient laboratory results, patient clinical outcomes, mass vaccination results, and social network analysis results.

Data from laboratory-based research activities can be stored in LabKey [6]. Data from patient-oriented research can be stored in REDCap [7], another secure, web-based clinical data management system [7]. Data from population-based research activities will be housed on numerous platforms due to the expected variety of file types (e.g., Microsoft Office formats, flash video, .mp4 video, .mp3 audio) (Figure 4.13).

A key aspect of the integration of each of these data sources is the building of data adapters or middleware to provide the adequate data linkages, which can be accomplished by using the application programming interfaces (APIs) provided by REDCap [7] and the LabKey-based [6] end-to-end comprehensive informatics infrastructure. Where necessary, patient clinical data and related laboratory research data will be linked

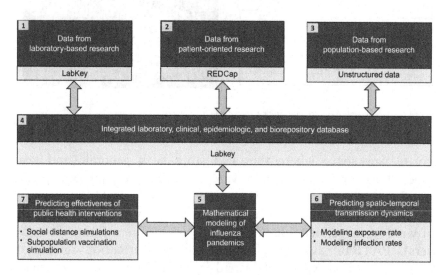

Figure 4.13 Example of data integration infrastructure for an influenza modeling project.

via a common subject identifier to support correlating laboratory-based, patient-oriented, and population-based research data.

Data Quality Control. Data quality control comprises four types of controls: database integrity, query response time controls, link integrity controls, and content accuracy controls. Database integrity begins with data loading controls. We will employ checksums on source files, comparisons of number of records in source file versus loaded to database, checks on required fields, and other referential integrity checks. Query response times will be monitored using built-in database diagnostics to collect performance data, analyze bottlenecks, and correct problems before they adversely impact users. Link integrity will be maintained using a tool such as GNU Wget to generate administrative reports on broken links. Cyberinfrastructure for immunoinformatics research should accommodate at least the minimal standard set of metadata for a particular type of experiment, for example, Minimum Information About a Proteomics Experiment (MIAPE) [8] for mass spectrometry and Minimum Information About a Flow Cytometry Experiment (MIFlowCyt) [9] for flow cytometry.

Standards Compliance. Adherence to data standards is a requisite for meaningful and successful data sharing and experiment reproducibility. Currently, the experimental approaches and technologies utilized by the immunology, natural product, biochemical research community generate datasets that range from the more traditional assays to measure immune responses (i.e., ELISA, ELISPOT, flow cytometry, immunophenotyping), to high-throughput screening of phenotypes (i.e., cytokine arrays, RNA-seq, proteomic or lipidomic analysis). The cyberinfrastructure for connecting data and modeling should implement a three-way standardization process based on (1) minimum information checklists, (2) data formats (syntax), and (3) controlled vocabularies and ontologies (semantics). This standardization process will guide the design of metadata templates for data submission.

Due to the numerous advantages of RNA-seq over microarray-based platforms for transcriptome characterization, large-scale projects such as The Cancer Genome Atlas (TCGA), TARGET, and the Cancer Genome Characterization Initiative have now mostly switched to RNA-seq for transcriptome profiling. However, the varieties of NGS technologies continue to shape their development and no universal standards have been established yet. NGS protocols should follow

Encyclopedia of DNA Elements (ENCODE) Consortium recommendations, such as "Standards, Guidelines and Best Practices for RNA-Seq 2010/2011" [10] and comply with the requirements of NCBI Gene Expression Omnibus (GEO).

Biomodels.net Submission. Published models will be uploaded to the Biomodels.net database. These models will be immediately available in the noncurated branch and will be curated by the Biomodels.net team and moved to the curated branch.

Model Standards. Standards such the Systems Biology Markup Language (SBML) should be considered to disseminate our models. There is a need to actively participate in the standards community to improve existing standards as well as to develop new standards when appropriate. There is an urgent need for a standard for encoding AGMs to facilitate exchange.

Data in NuML Format. The specification of the Numerical Markup Language (NuML), which has been derived from Systems Biology Result Markup Language (SBRML) format, has been finalized. An open-source support library should be developed for immunoinformatics projects.

Repository Data Interoperability. After data quality control and standard compliance, we will share the data through various repositories. Immunology raw and analyzed data will be shared through IMMPORT, a portal for immunology data sharing. Gene expression data will be deposited in GEO [11]. The metabolomics experiments and data will be deposited to Metabolights [12]. Models will be shared through the biomodels repository [13]. Compound library can be uploaded in PubChem [14], an open repository that enables identification of biological activities of small molecules. It contains three related databases: BioAssay, Compound, and Substance databases. BioAssay database contains bioactivity screens of chemical substances and test results. Compound database contains unique chemical structures while Substance database contains sample descriptions. In addition to depositing our results to PubChem, we will further work with PubChem datasets through Java API [15] and explore novel data-mining cheminformatics tools and virtual screening algorithms that are being developed [16–18] to further our understanding at a global level.

CONCLUDING REMARKS

We have presented the cyberinfrastructure required for immunoinformatics research connecting seamlessly experimental and computational immunology research. This infrastructure enables the MIEP team to investigate immunological processes at the system level and accelerate the development of information processing representations of the immune system. The systems approach enables us to produce high-quality, reproducible research results in an efficient way. The bioinformatics infrastructure in MIEP is constantly evolving to adapt for new experimental and computational technologies to keep the team competitive with the ultimate goal to connect fundamental immunological discoveries with accelerating the path to cures for human diseases.

ACKNOWLEDGMENTS

This work was supported in part by National Institute of Allergy and Infectious Diseases Contract No. HHSN272201000056C to JBR and funds from the Nutritional Immunology and Molecular Medicine Laboratory (www.nimml.org).

APPENDIX: MIEP DATA UPLOADED TO IMMPORT

	Paper	MIEP Web Portal	ImmPort UPLOAD DATE	Public, Semi-public, Private
1	The role of peroxisome proliferator-activated receptor γ in immune responses to enteroaggregative *Escherichia coli* infection	Available	Publicly available in ImmPort	Public
	PLoS One 2013;8(2):e57812. doi:10.1371/journal.pone.0057812. Epub 2013 Feb 28. PMID: 23469071			
2	Predictive computational modeling of the mucosal immune responses during *Helicobacter pylori* infection	Available	Publicly available in ImmPort	Public
	PLoS One 8(9):e73365. doi:10.1371/journal.pone.0073365			
3	Modeling the role of peroxisome proliferator-activated receptor γ and microRNA-146 in mucosal immune responses to *Clostridium difficile*	Available	Publicly available in ImmPort	Public
	PLoS One 2012;7(10):e47525. doi:10.1371/journal.pone.0047525. Epub 2012 Oct 11. PMID: 23071818			

4	Enteroaggregative *Escherichia coli* (EAEC) strain in a novel weaned mouse model: exacerbation by malnutrition, biofilm as a virulence factor, and treatment by nitazoxanide	Available	Publicly available in ImmPort	Public
	J Med Microbiol 2013;62(6):896–905. Epub ahead of print. PMID: 23475903			
5	Systems modeling of molecular mechanisms controlling cytokine-driven CD4+ T cell differentiation and phenotype plasticity	Available	Publicly available in ImmPort	Public
	PLoS Comput Biol 2013;9(4):e1003027. doi:10.1371/journal.pcbi.1003027. PMID: 23592971			
6	*Helicobacter pylori* infection in a pig model is dominated by Th1 and cytotoxic immune responses	Available	Publicly available in ImmPort	Public
	Infect Immun 2013. Epub ahead of print			
7	A novel pig model of *Helicobacter pylori* infection demonstrating Th1 and cytotoxic T cell responses	Available	Publicly available in ImmPort	Public
	Gut Microbes 2014;5(3):357–62. doi:10.4161/gmic.28899. Epub 2014 Apr 22. PMID: 24755940			
8	IL-21 is critical for the maintenance of effector T helper 1 and T helper 17 responses during chronic *Helicobacter pylori* infection	Available	Publicly available in ImmPort	Public
	MBio 2014;5(4):e01243-14. doi:10.1128/mBio.01243-14. PMID: 25053783			

REFERENCES

[1] Florez LA, et al. CellPublisher: a web platform for the intuitive visualization and sharing of metabolic, signalling and regulatory pathways. Bioinformatics 2010;26(23):2997–9.

[2] LabKey-Corporation. LabKey Software. 2015 (cited 2015 7/29). Available from: https://labkey.com/.

[3] Hasan SMS, et al. CINET: A CyberInfrastructure for NETwork science. In: Proceedings of the 2012 IEEE 8th international conference on e-Science. IEEE Computer Society; 2012. p. 1–8.

[4] Abdelhamid S, et al. CINET 2.0: a CyberInfrastructure for NETwork science. In: e-Science 2014 IEEE 10th International Conference. 2014.

[5] Wattam AR, et al. PATRIC, the bacterial bioinformatics database and analysis resource. Nucleic Acids Res 2014;42(D1):D581–91.

[6] Nelson EK, et al. LabKey Server: an open source platform for scientific data integration, analysis and collaboration. BMC Bioinformatics 2011;12:71.

[7] Harris PA, et al. Research electronic data capture (REDCap)—a metadata-driven methodology and workflow process for providing translational research informatics support. J Biomed Inform 2009;42(2):377–81.

[8] Taylor CF, et al. The minimum information about a proteomics experiment (MIAPE). Nat Biotechnol 2007;25(8):887–93.

[9] Spidlen J, et al. Flow cytometry data standards. BMC Res Notes 2011;4:50.

[10] Consortium EP. A user's guide to the encyclopedia of DNA elements (ENCODE). PLoS Biol 2011;9(4):e1001046.

[11] Edgar R, Domrachev M, Lash AE. Gene Expression Omnibus: NCBI gene expression and hybridization array data repository. Nucleic Acids Res 2002;30(1):207–10.

[12] Haug K, et al. MetaboLights—an open-access general-purpose repository for metabolomics studies and associated meta-data. Nucleic Acids Res 2013;41(D1):D781–6.

[13] Le Novere N, et al. BioModels Database: a free, centralized database of curated, published, quantitative kinetic models of biochemical and cellular systems. Nucleic Acids Res 2006;34 (Suppl. 1):D689–91.

[14] Wang Y, et al. PubChem: a public information system for analyzing bioactivities of small molecules. Nucleic Acids Res 2009;37(Web Server issue):W623–33.

[15] Southern MR, Griffin PR. A Java API for working with PubChem datasets. Bioinformatics 2011;27(5):741–2.

[16] Xie XQ. Exploiting PubChem for virtual screening. Expert Opin Drug Discov 2010;5 (12):1205–20.

[17] Ingsriswang S, Pacharawongsakda E. sMOL Explorer: an open source, web-enabled database and exploration tool for Small MOLecules datasets. Bioinformatics 2007;23 (18):2498–500.

[18] Matlock MK, Zaretzki JM, Swamidass SJ. Scaffold network generator: a tool for mining molecular structures. Bioinformatics 2013;29(20):2655–6.

CHAPTER 5

Ordinary Differential Equations (ODEs) Based Modeling

Stefan Hoops[1], Raquel Hontecillas[1], Vida Abedi[1], Andrew Leber[1], Casandra Philipson[2], Adria Carbo[2], and Josep Bassaganya-Riera[1]

[1]Nutritional Immunology and Molecular Medicine Laboratory, Virginia Bioinformatics Institute, Virginia Tech, Blacksburg, VA, USA [2]Biotherapeutics Inc., Blacksburg, VA, USA

INTRODUCTION

Ordinary differential equations (ODEs) have been used extensively and successfully to model an array of biological systems such as modeling network of gene regulation [1], signaling pathways [2], or biochemical reaction networks [3]. Thus, ODE-based models can be used to study the dynamics of systems, and facilitate identification of limit cycles, investigation of robustness and fragility of system, or help in the study of bifurcation behavior.

Modeling Network of Gene Regulation

Using temporal data, Chen et al. [4] developed differential equation model to represent gene expression and could demonstrate that the method was able and sufficient to construct a model at the genome level with a small set of temporal data. The model incorporated both transcription and translation by kinetic equations with feedback loops from the translation products to transcription. In addition, degradation of proteins and mRNAs was also incorporated. In a subsequent work by Ando et al. [5], hybrid Evolutionary Modeling of Genetic Programming approach was used to build causal model of differential equation system from time series data for modeling gene regulatory networks. In that model, the behavior of genes was modeled using differential equations. Hence, given the success of ODE-based model in the field, a comparative study was performed by Polynikis et al. [6] to investigate differences between different ODE modeling approaches in gene regulatory networks. In that study, it was demonstrated

Computational Immunology: Models and Tools. DOI: http://dx.doi.org/10.1016/B978-0-12-803697-6.00005-9

(by using a model system) that different models could lead to conflicting conclusions concerning the existence and stability of equilibria and stable oscillatory behaviors. It is therefore important to, whenever possible, make well-established modeling approximations and constrain as they can influence the overall system dynamics (e.g., ensure that all concentrations have to be positive). For a more comprehensive review of the literature, the reader is referred to a recent review by Chai et al. [1].

Modeling Signaling Pathways

Alteration of signaling pathways can lead to complex and unwanted phenotypes. Modeling such pathways can help in the identification of key components and their temporal behavior in a systematic way. Complex intracellular signaling networks can lead to different cellular behavior, and in tightly regulated and well-orchestrated systems, even minor alteration can be detrimental to the organism. Today with the accessibility of large-scale dataset, it is possible to identify key components of signaling pathways in high-throughput screenings; however, it will be the modeling efforts (such as ODE-based modeling) that could significantly help identify connectivity, cross talk, and dynamics of these key elements. For a recent review article, the reader is referred to a review by Bachmann et al. [2]. Using literature and available databases, it is possible to build a schematic signaling or transcriptional pathway which can be translated to an ODE model (see Chapter 7). To achieve greater efficiency, the schematic model can be constructed in SBML-compliant format (using CellDesigner [7] software) and imported directly into COPASI [8], an open-source software tool that is SBML-compliant and provides practical user interface for ODE-based models. For practical examples using COPASI and CellDesigner the reader is referred to Chapter 9. Once the model is constructed, parameters will be estimated (see section on Parameter Estimation) and *in silico* experimentation can be designed to generate plausible new hypothesis.

Modeling Biochemical Reaction Networks

Mathematical modeling, such as ODE-based modeling approaches, can be valuable to enhance our mechanistic understanding that is meaningful from the vast amount of available data. In a conventional reductionist approach, individual species (such as proteins) are studied independently; however, to have systems-level understanding of the

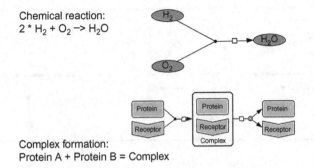

Chemical reaction:
$2 * H_2 + O_2 \rightarrow H_2O$

Complex formation:
Protein A + Protein B = Complex

Figure 5.1 Examples of biochemical processes.

overall process and discover emergent properties that arise from complex molecular-level interaction, it is fundamental to study species and their interactions simultaneously. Mathematical modeling can be of great tool toward this goal. At the first stage in the model development, there is a need to extract information and knowledge to build the model components. Once these components (such as proteins, enzymes, small molecules) are identified it is important to formulate their relationship using a mathematical formalism; for instance, ODE-based models or Boolean networks. Finally, once the model is constructed it will possible to estimate the parameters using in-house generated data or data from publications. A well-calibrated model can then be used to generate *in silico* experimentation and potentially novel hypothesis for further validation (Figure 5.1).

Modeling Multiple Scales

Modeling with ODEs is not limited to either biochemical processes or signaling pathways. An ODE model can span cell–cell interaction (including cell proliferation and cell death), intracellular process, and cytokine movement as seen in the *Clostridium difficile* host response model in Figure 5.2. The reader is referred to Chapter 9 for a step-by-step model development of the *C. difficile* host response.

ODE-Based Modeling Pipeline
Model Development

Before building a mathematical model, one needs to decide what the model shall describe and what the limits of the model shall be. For instance, it will not be appropriate to utilize quantum mechanics process involving electrons to describe a chemical reaction. Once the scope

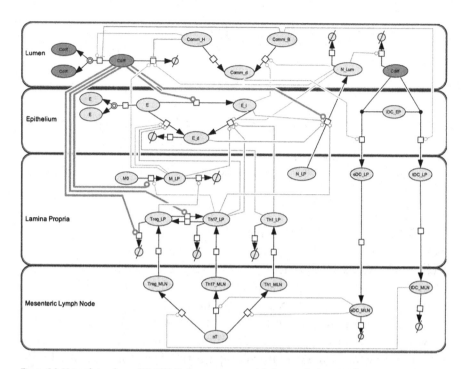

Figure 5.2 Network topology of C. difficile *host response model. Systems Biology Markup Language (SBML) compliant network of interactions between* C. difficile *and cellular immune components created in CellDesigner. Reaction modifiers connect cell nodes to reaction arrows with green an indication of activation and red of inhibition. Species consist of* C. difficile *(*Cdiff*), infection-exacerbating commensal bacteria (*Comm_H*), protective commensal bacteria (*Comm_B*), dead commensal bacteria (*Comm_d*), epithelial cells (*E*), inflamed epithelial cells (*E_i*), neutrophils (*N*), macrophages (*M*), dendritic cells (*tDC and eDC*), T cells (*nT, Treg, Th17, Th1*) existing in multiple compartments lumen (*Lum*), epithelium (*EP*), lamina propria (*LP*), and mesenteric lymph node (*MLN*). (For interpretation of the references to color in this figure legend, the reader is referred to the web version of this book.)*

of the model and its intended use is decided, one can start with the modeling process.

Interaction Network Creation. The first step of model development is to build an interaction network which depicts the components (variables) of the model and their interaction and transformations graphically. The tool we use for the graphical representation of the network is CellDesigner [9]. CellDesigner is an easy to use graphical tool (Figure 5.3) which is designed to create networks of biological interactions. The resulting graphical networks are understandable by experimentalists and mathematical modelers alike. Thus, CellDesigner facilitates the communication between the different team members. Furthermore, CellDesigner allows users to save the network in the Systems Biology Markup Language (SBML) [10], which subsequently

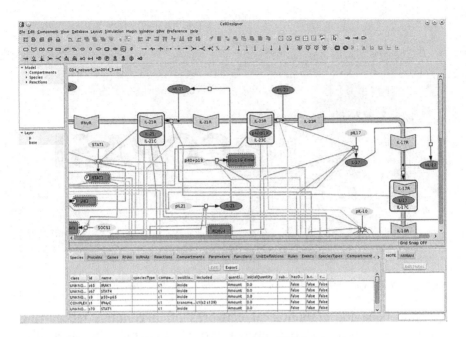

Figure 5.3 CellDesigner is a tool for creating interaction networks of biological processes.

allows modelers (including COPASI users) to easily move the model between a large set of tools. The knowledge for creating the interaction network is comprised of the expertise of the team members with domain knowledge, literature research, and experimental results (see Chapters 2, 3, and 7).

Adding Dynamics. Though the interaction network itself is valuable and its properties can be analyzed, computational biologists and modelers are usually more interested in the dynamic behavior of systems, that is, the change of the components over time. To add dynamic capabilities to the model, it is important to specify how fast the different processes are changing and how the participants influence this speed. The dynamic information is provided through kinetic rate laws. To add the rate laws to the interaction network, COPASI [8] can be used (Figure 5.4). The latter is a modeling and analysis tool for biochemical processes. COPASI is capable of importing the CellDesigner generated SBML file for faster and more efficient model development.

In general, three types of kinetic equations suffice to describe the dynamics of biological processes, namely: (1) mass action, (2) Michaelis–Menten, and (3) Hill equation kinetics [11]. Additionally,

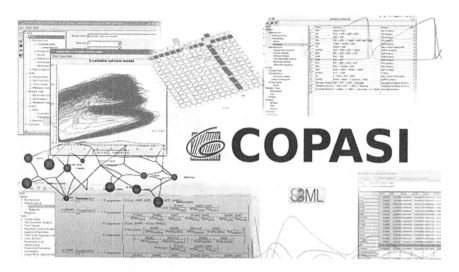

Figure 5.4 COPASI is a tool for modeling, simulation, and analysis of biochemical reaction networks.

dynamic behavior of biological networks often contains reoccurring wiring patterns known as "network motifs" that must be taken into consideration mathematically. One of the most integral network motifs is the feed-forward loop (FFL) that occurs during molecular cross talk [12]; for instance, molecule A regulates molecule B yet molecules A and B coregulate molecule C. FFLs are undoubtedly a common theme in our models and thus mathematics underlying macrophage signaling networks will adopt a combination of equations and parameters as justified herein.

The Hill equation is a sigmoidal function that easily represents switch mechanisms, such as transcription factor binding. The Hill model provides an advantage for estimating in a precise fashion to what extent positive or negative cooperativity between molecules exists [11]. Extensive studies have also demonstrated the benefits of the Hill equation for studying combinatorial regulation, especially those observed in FFLs [13], and therefore Hill equations will be used initially for characterizing cooperative roles among NLRs. Additionally, molecules that are regulated by several inputs (i.e., one gene jointly regulated by two transcription factors) may be calibrated given the assignment of a Hill equation. Mass action equations provide some advantages over Hill equations primarily related to their inherent ability to decipher mechanisms underlying molecular cooperativity rather than just positive or negative regulation (Hill model) [11]. Degradation rates and molecule transport are accurately represented by mass action equations. Mass action kinetics are also suitable for modeling multisite protein phosphorylation and are usually implemented in modeling complex biological systems due to their reliability in deterministic and stochastic simulations [14−16].

Model Calibration
Model development is followed by model calibration, where experimental data is often used to estimate the values of the kinetic parameters of the model. Some of the parameters may be known and can be determined by literature search. There are also databases that can be explored to extract parameter values; for instance, SABIO-RK [17,18] is a web-accessible database storing comprehensive information about biochemical reactions and their kinetic properties. However, even with availability of such databases, the value for some of the kinetic parameter cannot be determined. These parameters will be estimated for the model calibration process. In-house generated experimental data, or data from public repositories (like ImmPort and GEO), or literature search can be used for model calibration. The calibration is an optimization process which attempts to minimize the differences between the observed experimental data and the model simulation results by choosing the unknown parameters (Figure 5.5).

The calibration database may contain steady states, that is, endpoints of perturbation experiments or time course data. Since time course data describes the dynamic process in more detail, it is preferable for the parameter estimation process (see Chapter 7 on Time Series Analysis). Being able to generate time course data is extremely

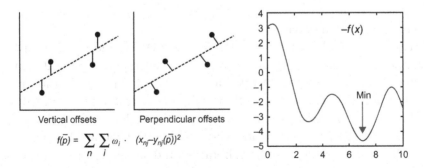

$$f(\bar{p}) = \sum_{n} \sum_{i} \omega_i \cdot (x_{ni} - y_{ni}(\bar{p}))^2$$

Figure 5.5 Parameter estimation attempts to find the set of parameters which minimizes the distance between the experimental data and the simulated values.

valuable, especially since such rich data can be particularly useful for model calibration process.

COPASI has built-in capabilities for the model calibration process. In fact, the software provides several optimization algorithms that modelers can utilize. The calibration database can be easily imported into COPASI and the objective function (see Figure 5.5) can be automatically generated. As a general guideline, the parameter estimation process can start with a global optimization algorithm such as Particle Swarm [19] or evolutionary algorithms [20]. Commonly we repeat this process multiple times to gain confidence in the solution. To refine the result local algorithm such as Levenberg–Marquardt [21,22] can be used.

To determine the confidence of parameters, the Sigma Point method [23] implemented in Condor-COPASI [24] can be utilized. Condor-COPASI is provided through bioinformatics infrastructure (see Chapter 4) utilizing VBI's high-performance computing (HPC) capabilities.

The main challenge of parameter estimation is due to the lack of sufficient experimental data. However, if the model is incorrect, either in its network structure or the chosen dynamics, it is nearly impossible to fit the (sometimes limited) experimental data independent of the number of unknown parameters contrary to the quote: "With four parameters I can fit an elephant, and with five I can make him wiggle his trunk" which is attributed to van Neumann. Please note that we are not necessarily interested in the "correct" parameters as long as the resulting model has predicting power. In essence, a model that can reproduce observed dynamic behavior can be used to generate novel hypothesis and be instrumental in knowledge discovery.

Deterministic Simulations
A calibrated model can be used for further analysis and *in silico* experimentation. When a model is calibrated, it can reproduce the dynamic behavior of all the experiments that were used for the calibration process. Using simulations, it will be possible to examine intermediate values and project long-term behavior of the system. COPASI can be used to perform the simulation very efficiently. Chapter 9 provides a step-by-step process of model calibration and simulation for three case studies. Nevertheless, for sake of clarity, the main steps are summarized here. In essence, *Time Course task* can be used on the calibrated

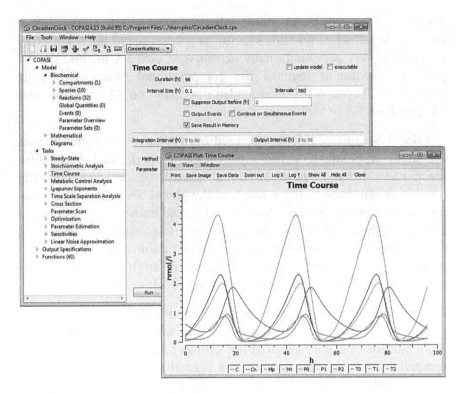

Figure 5.6 Time course simulation with COPASI.

mode to generate simulation; however, it will be important to select the duration for the simulation. Different simulation can be performed instantaneously for different initial conditions in order to study the system more closely; it is also possible to modify the system in unique ways to further enhance our understanding of the properties of the system, some of these interventions may not even be possible (or very time consuming) in a wet-lab setting (Figure 5.6).

Sensitivity Analysis

Sensitivity analysis (SA) is often employed to quantify the importance of each of the model's parameters on the behavior of the system. We can distinguish between local and global SA. A local SA addresses sensitivity relative to change of a single parameter value, while a global analysis examines sensitivity with regard to the entire parameter distribution. Whereas global SA focuses on the variance of model outputs and determines how input parameters influence the output parameters. It is a central tool in SA since it provides a quantitative and rigorous overview of how different inputs influence the output. Global SA is often preferred when possible, due to its greater detail but for a large system it is very computationally expensive. Local SA method can be preferred because it requires less computational power. Reader is referred to Chapter 6 for an extended discussion on SA of ABM, and Chapter 8 on SA of multiscale models.

Global Sensitivity [25] can be used even without the knowledge of the unknown parameters. This means it can be performed even before the model calibration process. Global SA can be used to reduce the number of parameters. If the result of the global SA is that a parameter does not influence the outcome, that is, the maximum or minimum change of the outcome is near zero. Since this result is independent from the setting of all parameters the studied parameters value is irrelevant and can be removed or be assigned an arbitrary value. Global SA can be performed with Condor-COPASI [24].

Local SA focuses more on a single input's behavior while other parts remain the same. It is narrow in this aspect as the effect of an input parameter is not measured for settings other than the base. Local sensitivity is nevertheless a great tool once the model is calibrated. It can be helpful in determining which parameter should be modified for the system to reproduce a desired outcome. Local SA can be performed in COPASI directly. In order to perform SA in COPASI, one has to select an outcome or desirable effect and provide a list of candidate parameters. COPASI will return a color-coded table that highlights which parameter influenced the outcome and in which direction.

COPASI provides scaled and unscaled results. Unscaled result presents the ratio of the absolute change of the effect to absolute change of the parameter or cause. Scaled result represents the ratio of the relative changes (Figure 5.7).

Model-Driven Hypothesis Generation

Generating model-driven hypothesis can be extremely powerful as it is very efficient and cost-effective to generate "what-if-scenarios" with the ODE-based models. Therefore, one should study possible interventions *in silico* to determine whether they have the desired (or nonintuitive) effects. Once such intervention candidate is found, the model can be used to help design the wet-lab experiment that can be most rewarding.

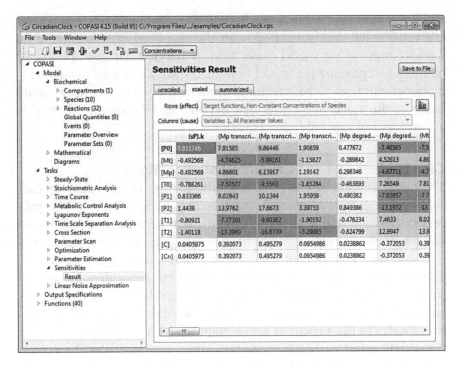

Figure 5.7 Scaled local sensitivity analysis result in COPASI. Intensive green values mean strong positive effect whereas intensive red values are strong negative effects, pale or white values indicate minor change. (For interpretation of the references to color in this figure legend, the reader is referred to the web version of this book.)

We used our comprehensive CD4+ T-cell differentiation model [26] to make experimental predictions focused on the role of transcription factor PPARγ, peroxisome proliferator-activated receptor gamma, in controlling the plasticity between Th17 and Treg subsets. In an *in silico* knockout of PPARγ, the model predicted an increased prevalence of Th17 cells. The prediction was validated with an *in vivo* model of experimental colitis. In the PPARγ null mice, the percentage of Treg cells was decreased and the percentage of Th17 cells was increased with respect to the wild-type mice. Additionally, *in silico* experimentation displayed the effect of stimulating PPARγ in switching a Th17 phenotype to a Treg phenotype and how various levels of activated PPARγ would predispose a cell to a phenotype. These predictions were also validated experimentally using administration of a PPARγ-activator pioglitazone to mice with experimentally induced colitis. This initial utilization of the computational modeling predictions displays the value of these methods in the generation of hypotheses and highly focused experimental designs.

Please note that even if the hypothesis generated with a model is not verified the data generated from the suggested experiment can be used to improve the model calibration. If the new data can no longer be fitted by changing the model parameters, we know that the model is incorrect and need to be structurally modified until we can successfully calibrate the model and create new hypothesis. "Essentially, all models are wrong, but some are useful" [27].

Case Studies: CD4+ T-Cell Differentiation Model

The differentiation of CD4+ T cells into mature phenotypes is dependent on a multitude of molecule types and signaling pathways. This process is generally initiated with the activation of a naïve T cell by an antigen-presenting cell. Upon activation, the fate of the cellular phenotype becomes largely controlled by the extracellular cytokine milieu. The binding of these cytokines to their respective receptors on the cell surface begins a cascade of enzymatic events resulting in the phosphorylation of STAT proteins. In turn, the phosphorylated STAT protein translocates to the nucleus at which point the STAT is able to activate a transcription factor. The transcription factor then regulates the expression of genes either through activation or inhibition, which ultimately determines the functionality and phenotype of the cell. However, despite historical views that the differentiation of CD4+ T cells is a rigid process from naïve cells to a terminal cell type, recent studies have proven that flexibility and plasticity exist throughout and even after the differentiation process. The development of an ODE-based model describing the differentiation of Th1, Th2, Th17, and iTreg cells has been a valuable resource in the understanding of both the plasticity of CD4+ T-cell phenotypes and the impact of the various factors on these differentiation events. In combination with mouse studies, we have gained mechanistic insights into the modulation of CD4+ T-cell differentiation in the gastrointestinal mucosa (Figure 5.8).

A thorough literature search was used to generate an initial prototype of the model network, which was further expanded based on hypotheses and new findings to encompass over 50 reactions and greater than 90 model species. To define this network, a system of 60 ordinary differential equations was used including numerous mathematical functions to describe mass action, activation and inhibition, and reversible and irreversible reactions. Using data obtained through the search and our own laboratory-generated data, an expansive

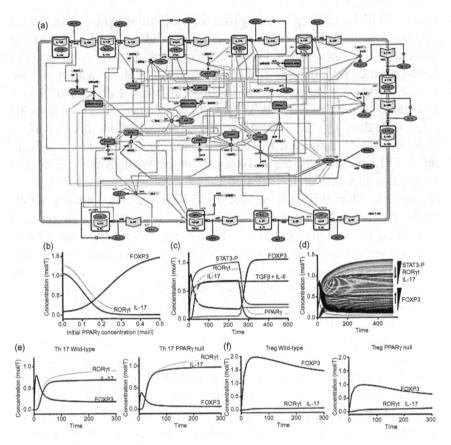

Figure 5.8 (a) CellDesigner-based CD4+ T-cell network model illustrating pathways involved in CD4+ T-cell differentiation into T helper (Th)1, Th2, Th17, and iTreg. Revised network model including the externalization of cytokines. (b) Scan illustrating the effects of PPARγ activation on Th17 cells in silico. (c) Time course illustrating the effects of PPARγ activation on Th17 cells, including down-modulation of IL-17, STAT3, RORγt and upregulation of FOXP3 in a differentiated Th17 cell following PPARγ activation. (d) Time course and scan combination of Th17 following PPAR γ activation to assess changes in IL-17, STAT3, RORγt, and FOXP3 over time. (e and f) Graphs illustrate the impact of in silico deletion of PPARγ on iTreg and Th17 phenotypes. All versions of the CD4 + T-cell network model are available at the MIEP website under Modeling, Models, CD4+ T-cell differentiation model (http://www.modelingimmunity.org/modeling/copasi/copasi-cd4-t-cell-differentiation).

calibration data set was created comprised of a variety of *in vivo* knockout studies and *in vitro* stimulation conditions, among other data. With the algorithms present within COPASI, the model parameters were estimated and optimized to best represent the known data. Afterward, the model was able to accurately display preferential differentiation in stimulating conditions specific to each of the four subsets.

The first use of the model to make experimental predictions focused on the role of transcription factor PPARγ in controlling the plasticity between Th17 and Treg subsets. In a scan of initial values of activated PPAR-γ, higher initial amounts switched the differentiation prediction from a Th17 state to an iTreg state (Figure 5.8(b)). Alternatively, scan parameter values controlling PPAR-γ activation within a time course simulation displayed a similar result with decreases of Th17-associated molecules IL17, ROR-γt and phosphorylated STAT3 occurring at higher levels of PPAR-γ activation. Additionally, *in silico* experimentation displayed the effect of stimulating PPAR-γ in switching a Th17 phenotype to an iTreg phenotype through the creation of an event which artificially elevated the amount of activated PPAR-γ in the system. After this increase, the Th17 state that was initially generated switches to the one dominated by iTreg differentiation (Figure 5.8 (c)). These predictions were also validated experimentally using administration of a PPAR-γ-activator pioglitazone to mice with experimentally induced colitis. Finally in an *in silico* knockout of PPAR-γ, the model predicted an increased prevalence of Th17 cells and decreased prevalence of iTreg cells (Figure 5.8(e) and (f)). This prediction was also validated with an *in vivo* model of experimental colitis. In the PPAR-γ null mice, the percentage of Treg cells was decreased and the percentage of Th17 cells was increased with respect to the wild-type mice. This initial utilization of the computational modeling predictions displays the value of these methods in the generation of hypotheses and highly focused experimental designs. The CD4+ T-cell differentiation model was further used to elucidate a mechanism of IL-21 in the context of chronic *Helicobacter pylori* infection. Prior to experimentation in this field, the model was first recalibrated using *H. pylori* specific data in a similar manner to the generalized initial calibration. SA on the model was conducted to identify important effects of IL-21 on other molecules in the system. In particular, the analysis suggested that the largest impact of IL-21was on the Th17-associated molecules IL-17, ROR-γt, and phosphorylated STAT3. An increase in IL-21 would indicate an increase in those three proteins. The analysis also showed that an increase in IL-21 would also have a similar positive effect on Th1-associated molecules phosphorylated STAT1, T-bet, and IFN-γ while having a negative effect on Treg-associated FOXP3 and IL-10. Consequentially, when an *in silico* knockout of IL-21 was conducted, a decrease in both Th17 and Th1 was seen. The *in silico* results compared favorably to the percent change seen experimentally in IL-21 knockout mice challenged with *H. pylori*. These results suggest that IL-21 could be a crucial determinant for chronic inflammation during

H. pylori colonization. In this case, the computational model displayed an ability to identify a highly important node within the system able to cause a large experimental impact *in vivo*.

CONCLUDING REMARKS

With higher computational power and HPC capabilities (see Chapter 4), modeling can be transformative especially if applied in a multiscale setting. Multiscale modeling approaches use modeling at different levels (from genes to tissue levels) and attempt to provide a more comprehensive view of the overall systems dynamic whenever there is adequate experimental data for model calibration and model testing. Chapter 8 focuses on multiscale modeling more broadly with an additional case study. ODE-based models are used to describe parts of the multiscale model.

ACKNOWLEDGMENTS

This work was supported in part by National Institute of Allergy and Infectious Diseases Contract No. HHSN272201000056C to JBR and funds from the Nutritional Immunology and Molecular Medicine Laboratory (www.nimml.org).

REFERENCES

[1] Chai LE, et al. A review on the computational approaches for gene regulatory network construction. Comput Biol Med 2014;48:55−65.

[2] Bachmann J, et al. Predictive mathematical models of cancer signalling pathways. J Intern Med 2012;271(2):155−65.

[3] Neelamegham S, Liu G. Systems glycobiology: biochemical reaction networks regulating glycan structure and function. Glycobiology 2011;21(12):1541−53.

[4] Chen T, He HL, Church GM. Modeling gene expression with differential equations. Pac Symp Biocomput 1999;29−40.

[5] Ando S, Sakamoto E, Iba H. Evolutionary modeling and inference of gene network. Inf Sci 2002;145(3−4):237−59.

[6] Polynikis A, Hogan SJ, di Bernardo M. Comparing different ODE modelling approaches for gene regulatory networks. J Theor Biol 2009;261(4):511−30.

[7] Funahashi A, et al. CellDesigner 3.5: a versatile modeling tool for biochemical networks. Proc IEEE 2008;96(8):1254−65.

[8] Hoops S, et al. COPASI—a COmplex PAthway SImulator. Bioinformatics 2006;22 (24):3067−74.

[9] Funahashi A, et al. CellDesigner: a process diagram editor for gene-regulatory and biochemical networks. Biosilico 2003;1(5):159−62.

[10] Hucka M, et al. The Systems Biology Markup Language (SBML): a medium for representation and exchange of biochemical network models. Bioinformatics 2003;19(4):524–31.

[11] Radivoyevitch T. Mass action models versus the Hill model: an analysis of tetrameric human thymidine kinase 1 positive cooperativity. Biol Direct 2009;4:49.

[12] Le DH, Kwon YK. A coherent feedforward loop design principle to sustain robustness of biological networks. Bioinformatics 2013;29(5):630–7.

[13] Mangan S, Alon U. Structure and function of the feed-forward loop network motif. Proc Natl Acad Sci USA 2003;100(21):11980–5.

[14] Barik D, et al. A model of yeast cell-cycle regulation based on multisite phosphorylation. Mol Syst Biol 2010;6:405.

[15] Qu Z, Weiss JN, MacLellan WR. Regulation of the mammalian cell cycle: a model of the G1-to-S transition. Am J Physiol Cell Physiol 2003;284(2):C349–64.

[16] Kapuy O, et al. Bistability by multiple phosphorylation of regulatory proteins. Prog Biophys Mol Biol 2009;100(1–3):47–56.

[17] Wittig U, et al. SABIO-RK: integration and curation of reaction kinetics data. Heidelberg, Germany: Springer; 2006.

[18] Li P, et al. Systematic integration of experimental data and models in systems biology. BMC Bioinformatics 2010;11.

[19] Kennedy J, Eberhart R. Particle swarm optimization. In: Proceedings of IEEE international conference on neural networks, New York, NY; 1995. p. 39–43.

[20] Baeck T, Schwefel H-P. An overview of evolutionary algorithms for parameter optimization. Evol Comput 1993;1(1):1–23.

[21] Levenberg K. A method for the solution of certain non-linear problems in least squares. Quar J Appl Math 01/1944; 2(2):164–8.

[22] Marquardt DW. An algorithm for least-squares estimation of nonlinear parameters. J Soc Ind Appl Math 1963;11(2):431–41.

[23] Van Der Merwe R, Wan EA, Julier S. Sigma-point Kalman filters for nonlinear estimation and sensor-fusion: applications to integrated navigation. In: Proceedings of the AIAA guidance, navigation & control conference. 2004. pp. 16–19.

[24] Kent E, Hoops S, Mendes P. Condor-COPASI: high-throughput computing for biochemical networks. BMC Syst Biol 2012;6:91.

[25] Sahle S, et al. A new strategy for assessing sensitivities in biochemical models. Philos Trans A Math Phys Eng Sci 2008;366(1880):3619–31.

[26] Carbo A, et al. Systems modeling of molecular mechanisms controlling cytokine-driven CD4+ T cell differentiation and phenotype plasticity. PLoS Comput Biol 2013;9(4): e1003027.

[27] Box GE, Draper NR. Empirical model-building and response surfaces, vol. 424. New York, NY: Wiley; 1987.

CHAPTER 6

Agent-Based Modeling and High Performance Computing

Maksudul Alam[4], Vida Abedi[1], Josep Bassaganya-Riera[1], Katherine Wendelsdorf[2], Keith Bisset[4], Xinwei Deng[3], Stephen Eubank[4], Raquel Hontecillas[1], Stefan Hoops[1], and Madhav Marathe[4]

[1]Nutritional Immunology and Molecular Medicine Laboratory, Virginia Bioinformatics Institute, Virginia Tech, Blacksburg, VA, USA [2]Applied Advanced Genomics, QIAGEN, Redwood City, CA, USA [3]Department of Statistics, Virginia Tech, Blacksburg, VA, USA [4]Network Dynamics and Simulation Science Laboratory, Virginia Bioinformatics Institute, Virginia Tech, Blacksburg, VA, USA

INTRODUCTION AND BASIC DEFINITIONS

Current experimental techniques are limited in their ability to quantitatively manipulate immune responses to pathogens in a controlled manner in animal models and to trace events at the tissue level confidently back to specific cellular level interactions and molecular mechanisms. In a mathematical model, one can test whether mechanisms seen in the experimental context *in vivo* or *in vitro* are plausible explanations for phenomena observed at the clinical level. Such a tool is at the very heart of translational research. Modeling Immunity to Enteric Pathogens (MIEP) (http://www.modelingimmunity.org/) has created large-scale high-resolution models of immune responses at the cellular level that realize this exciting potential. Building a computational model to understand and provide insights into the time-varying behavior of a biological system is valuable, especially when such model takes into account many different factors, such as availability and types of data, the scales (molecular to tissue level), and computational resources. It is also important to use the appropriate modeling formalism, such as equation-based or agent-based models (ABMs) or an integrated system where multiple modeling formalism is unified to function together (see Chapter 8 for multiscale modeling (MSM)).

Computational Immunology: Models and Tools. DOI: http://dx.doi.org/10.1016/B978-0-12-803697-6.00006-0

Equation-based models, such as ODEs (ordinary differential equations), PDEs (partial differential equations), and SDEs (stochastic differential equations) are frequently used to model biological systems at various levels of complexity (see Chapter 5). These types of models can capture quantitative spatiotemporal system behavior. The models have been the workhorse of mathematical biologists. The models have been immensely successful and have been used by researchers to gain important insights in systems biology (e.g., see Chapter 5 and the references therein). Despite their simplicity and effectiveness, developing good equation-based models remain challenging. First, developing efficient solutions to large ODEs and PDEs is often computationally challenging due to their size, especially when biologists seek to better understand multiscale phenomenon at higher levels of resolutions. Furthermore, since ODEs are typically used to model entire populations rather than individual entities, stochasticity must be incorporated (SDE-based models) at the population level. However, the population-level consequences of individual interactions are not always apparent; therefore, the population-level description of stochastic effects arising from variations at the individual level requires prior knowledge of system's overall behavior.

ABMs serve as a natural computational representation when there is enough information about the behavior of individual entities (in isolation) and their interactions with (small) number of other entities. For instance, there is a large body of *in vitro* studies of T-cell behavior and differentiation that is suitable for agent-based modeling. ABMs are most appropriate when the focus of the study is on emergence of complexity, and the model is based on a limited number of species. Using ABMs, it is generally easy to include qualitative dynamical constraints; it is also practical to model local individual–individual interactions that are influenced by spatial proximity, thus integrating context specificity into the model without the need for added computational resources.

In essence, an ABM comprises agents and their interactions. For example, agents can (i) have properties to represent different entity states (e.g., sex, genotypes, size, and color), (ii) be assigned to specific locations and move spatially, (iii) interact with other agents and the environment, and (iv) be represented in a hierarchical structure. An ABM is capable of modeling multiscale and highly complex biological phenomena; furthermore, ABMs can also integrate multiple modeling technologies. Further detail on MSM using ABM can be found in Chapter 8.

ABMs are sometimes considered less rigorous than equation-based models; however, this is not the case. In essence, the formal theory of ABMs and the rationale to develop such models is discussed further in Refs. [1–4].

In this chapter, we introduce ENISI a high performance computing (HPC)–based ABM designed to study the inflammatory and regulatory immune pathways initiated by interactions among microbes and immune cells in the gut [1,2]. ENISI can represent various regulatory and effector cell types and their interactions in great detail. Individual cells, along with their movement through different tissues, and the probabilistic outcomes of cell–cell interaction are modeled using scripting language. ENISI simulates the models using scalable parallel algorithms and implementations for HPC-based systems. ENISI is capable of scaling to 10^7 individual cells.

RELATED WORK

ABMs have been used successfully to study complex systems in biology [5]. Parunak et al. [6] compared ABMs with equation-based models. Materi et al. [7] discussed computational modeling techniques, including ODEs, PDEs, and ABMs, and tools used in drug discovery and development. Various models of mucosal infection captured the aspects of inflammatory and regulatory immune pathways [8–11]. These models have provided insight into mechanisms of clinical symptoms as well as pathogen persistence.

Mathematical models have been employed to capture the dynamics of the immune system. Most of the models are based on differential equations. ODEs have been used to model immune cells in Refs. [12–16]. ODEs are used because of their relatively simpler mathematical formalism and computational efficiency.

Delay differential equations (DDE) have been used to capture the delayed responses of biological systems in Refs. [17,18]. PDEs are also used in Refs. [13,19], which take into account cell age and location.

These models are deterministic and do not capture the stochastic behavior of cells. An SDE model was also proposed in Ref. [20].

Agent-based modeling provides an alternative approach to model the immune systems with a population of distinct interacting agents representing cells with appropriate set of rules, and the outcomes are observed at the system scale. ABMs have been used widely in areas such as computer science [21], economics, biology, ecology, and social phenomena. The intrinsically spatial component [22] and the fact that the system can easily integrate different kinds of experimental data into one *in silico* experimental system [23] make ABMs a popular choice (see Refs. [23−25] for a detailed and comprehensive discussion on this topic). Aspects of the inflammatory and regulatory immune pathway models presented here have been shown in previous models of mucosal infection [8−11] to yield insight into mechanisms of clinical symptoms as well as pathogen persistence. Many studies have successfully used ABMs to simulate the dynamics of inflammation [26−30]. With the exponential growth of technological and computational power in the past decade, ABMs have become even more popular. For a comprehensive review of agent-based modeling applied to immune systems and its limitations and challenges, please see Ref. [24].

Several ABMs have been developed for modeling immune systems in the last two decades including AbAIS (Agent-based Artificial IS) [31], CAFISS [32], ImmSim [33], ImmSim3 [34], C-ImmSim [35], ParImm [35], ImmunoGrid [36], Rhapsody [37,38], SIS [39], SIMMUNE [40], NFSim [41], BIS [42], and the work reported in Ref. [43]. Comprehensive surveys can be found in [24,25,44]. REPAST [45] is another advanced, free, and open-source Java-based agent-based modeling platform [46,47]. There are also hybrid models, ABMs combined with delay differential equation models (ABM-DDE), which attempt to investigate dynamics over a wide range of parameters [48]. The latter decouple the agent interactions from the dynamics of the system in order to better understand the unique features of the biological system and predict conditions that will promote certain phenotypic behavior.

In Ref. [49], Marino et al. developed a multiorgan hybrid model of granuloma formation and T-cell priming in tuberculosis. The hybrid model was composed of an ABM for the lung compartment and a nonlinear system of ODEs representing the lymph node (LN) compartment. The computational model was instrumental in analyzing the protective mechanisms by providing some evidence that effector CD4+ T cells may be able to rescue the system from a persistent infection and lead to clearance once a granuloma is fully formed. This finding can be used as an immunotherapy strategy for latently infected individuals. An [50] modeled the Toll-like receptor 4 (TLR4) signaling and the inflammatory response and tolerance using ABM framework. The ABM incorporates an abstracted molecular "event" rule system with a spatially explicit representation of the relationship between signaling and synthetic compounds. This model was able to capture the main dynamics of the TLR4 signal transduction cascade, including stochastic signal behavior, dose-dependent response, negative feedback control, and pre-conditioning effects.

These simulators place an emphasis on rules governing cell–cell contacts and signaling interactions allowing one to enter complicated functions for these mechanisms. They, therefore, provide the useful capability of incorporating complex mathematical models for receptor–ligand interactions and phenotype differentiation into cell contact networks. However, it is not clear how these implementations scale to more complex systems and larger numbers of cells in a network nor how easy they are for those who are not experts in computing to use. For example, Rhapsody has been shown to simulate up to 10^4 individuals efficiently [37,38]. SIMMUNE is the most sophisticated modeling environment in terms of making the system user friendly. It can handle 5×10^5 cells per processor [40] but requires substantial computing. A recent version of SIMMUNE is substantially more expressive, has an improved graphical interface, and focuses on allowing biologists to interact with the modeling environment [51,52].

All the models mentioned above are based on sequential programming model. In contrast to those models, the work on parallel ABM for immune system modeling is not extensive. C-ImmSim [35] and ImmunoGrid [36] are two well-known parallel simulators for modeling the immune system that can scale to reasonably large system sizes. SIS is also supposed to scale large systems, but details about this scaling are not clear from the published work. These simulators are discrete in space and time and use an underlying geometry to represent spatial interactions.

The ENISI model is unique in its scope and approach. The model incorporates regulatory mechanisms of both adaptive and innate immunity, multilocation migration of cells, and cross talk between antigen-presenting cells and T cells. It is an ABM that explicitly represents each participating cell of the immune pathway, their movement across compartments, proliferation when appropriate, and their differentiation. This facilitates mapping model parameter specifications and predictions to laboratory techniques, such as flow cytometry, which manipulate specific cell populations. We previously implemented a larger scale version of the model, encompassing these aspects, as a system of ODEs. Simulations based on this initial version identified a relationship between the effector CD4+ T helper cells (Th) and classically activated M1 macrophage concentrations in the lamina propria (LP) and chronic epithelial damage [53]. In addition, we have successfully modeled the intracellular pathways controlling CD4+ T cell differentiation based on the external cytokine milieu [54] as well as the cellular interactions underlying host responses to *Helicobacter pylori* infection by using ODE and agent-based approaches [54]. However, ODEs can only capture the dynamics of each cell population as a whole. Hence, this work builds on previous studies from our group [55] and identified a relationship between M1 and Th levels and epithelial damage, which could not be easily identified using ODEs. An additional drawback of the ODE representation is that it assumes deterministic average behavior by each individual cell. SDEs can alleviate some of these issues, but the computational complexity of solving them grows considerably and defeats the purpose of using simple differential equation-based models. ABMs provide a natural alternative by incorporating stochasticity in the models.

The ENISI model is an extension of the interacting state machine models or ABMs. A key aspect of these models is a procedural and interactive (also known as mechanistic, algorithmic, and executable) view of the underlying systems [56]. In this view, components of the system interact locally with other components and the behavior of individual objects is described procedurally as a function of the internal state and the local interactions. This agent-based approach allows incorporation of spatial effects and randomness of cell–cell and cell–bacteria contact. In the case of colonic inflammation spawned by a small number of pathogens, such randomness is believed to significantly affect the outcome of the system, and, therefore, an ABM is an appropriate representation [24]. This also creates a foundation for composed (also known as "emergent") properties such as bacterial strain evolution and changes in microflora demographics as the model is elaborated and the simulator extended. However, the drawback to such methods is that they are often not scalable due to limitations of computation power.

Scalability is important when seeking to reproduce emergent tissue-level phenomena by simulating individual cell interactions. Large-scale models are necessary because the purpose of immune simulators is to reproduce dynamics in a true *in vivo* system where immune cell concentrations can reach 10^8/ml [57]. It may not be sufficient to simulate the dynamics of a small sample and extrapolate results to the entire organ. The scaling and parallel efficiency achieved by ENISI is one of its distinguishing features.

TECHNICAL IMPLEMENTATION OF ENISI

MIEP (www.modelingimmunity.org) has developed an integrated modeling and *in silico* experimentation environment for supporting the proposed goals. One example is ENISI, an HPC-based tool for modeling the mucosal immune responses with the ability to simulate *in silico* experiments from signaling pathways to tissue-level events. The *in silico* experimentation environment is intended to provide novel ways for scientist to study the immune system by making HPC-based solutions easily accessible and consists of the following components.

1. High-resolution scalable models of complex immunological systems;
2. Service-oriented architecture and delivery mechanism for facilitating the use of these models by domain experts;
3. Scalable methods for visual and data analytics to support analysts.

The model and service architecture is based on a *mathematical theory of coevolving systems*. The mathematical theory plays a crucial role here. It underwrites the development of efficient HPC-oriented models, provides a formal specification for the service architecture, and is the basis of the service delivery and analytic framework. The mathematical theory and the proposed interaction-based models seek to address the complicated *interplay* between the three components that contribute to irreducibility of such systems: (*i*) individual behaviors of agents (cells, organs, and molecules), (*ii*) unstructured and heterogeneous multiscale interaction networks, and (*iii*) the dynamical processes on these networks.

FORMAL REPRESENTATION OF ENISI

Interaction-Based Approach for Modeling Gut Mucosa: Coevolving Graphical Discrete Dynamical Systems (CGDDS)

Our ABMs are built on rigorous mathematical foundations—one of the unique aspects of our work. These are called graphical discrete dynamical systems [58,59]. The mathematical model consists of two parts: (i) a coevolving graphical discrete dynamical system framework (CGDDS) that captures the coevolution of system dynamics, interaction network, and individual object behavior and (ii) a partially observable Markov decision process that captures various control and optimization problems formulated on the phase space of this dynamical system. A CGDDS consists of a dynamic graph $G_t(V_t, E_t)$ in which vertices represents individual objects (agents) and edges represent a causal relationship that is usually local, a set of *local state machines* (automata), one for each vertex specifying the behavior of the agents, and a set of *update functions*, one per edge that describes how an edge can be modified as a function of the state of its end points. The state and behavioral changes of individual objects are a function of their internal state and its interaction with neighboring agents. These neighbors change over time and space, and thus the model needs to explicitly represent this network evolution.

Let $V = (v_1, v_2, \ldots, v_n)$ represents the set of immune cells or bacteria and $S = (S_1, S_2, \ldots, S_m)$ be the set of all possible states (phenotypes) that the cells can take. Also define $s_t(v) \in S$ as the state of any vertex $v \in V$ at time t. For each vertex (cell) v, g denotes the update function that takes as input the state of the vertex $s_t(v)$ at time t and returns the set of edges that v will be adjacent to in a given period of time. In other words, g captures the time-varying edges at $t + 1$ in the graph. For each vertex $v \in V$, let f be the function representing the local state machine. The function f takes as input the state of the vertex $s_t(v)$ at time t, the states of other vertices of the edges incident on v, and results the state $s_{t+1}(v)$ at time $t + 1$ as output. If vertices $(v_1, v_2, \ldots, v_k)$ are adjacent to vertex v, we can define the state transition function f for v as:

$$s_{t+1}(v) = f(s_t(v), s_t(v_1), s_t(v_2), \ldots, s_t(v_k))$$

At any time t, the configuration $\zeta(t)$ of a CGDDS is defined as a vector $(s_t(v_1), s_t(v_2), \ldots, s_t(v_n))$, the states of all vertices. The time evolution of a CGDDS is represented by the sequence of successive configuration changes of the dynamic network. The ABM simulation is

Algorithm 6.1 Pseudo-code describing ENISI execution as formalized using CGDDS

for $t = 0$ **to** T **do**
    Compute the interaction graph G_t using function g
    for each vertex v **do**
    Compute $s_t(v)$ using state update function f

performed by evaluating the dynamic graph for a given number of time steps T as shown in Algorithm 6.1.

CGDDS serve as a bridge between mathematical simulation theory and HPC design and implementation. Similar to state charts and other formal models [56], they can be used for formal specification, design, and analysis of multiscale biological and social systems. CGDDS extend the algebraic theory of dynamical systems in two important ways. First, we pass from extremely general structural and analytical properties of composed local maps to issues of provable implementation of sequential dynamical systems in computing architectures and to specification of interacting local symbolic procedures generally. This is related to successive reductions of CGDDS to procedural primitives, which leads to a notion of CGDDS-based distributed simulation compilers with provable simulated dynamics (e.g., for massively parallel or grid computation). Second, the aggregate behavior of iterated compositions of local maps that comprise a CGDDS can be understood as a (specific) simulated algorithm together with its associated and inherent computational complexity. We have called this the algorithmic semantics of a CGDDS (equivalently, the algorithmic semantics of a dynamical system or a simulation). It is particularly important to view a composed dynamical system as computing a specifiable algorithm with provable time and space performance. Basic results on the mathematical and computational aspects of CGDDS can be found in a series of articles [58,60,61]. CGDDS has been applied to a wide range of distributed dynamical systems such as social contact graphs [59], urban traffic and transportation [62], epidemics [58], dynamics of biological systems [63], and gene annotation [64]. We have successfully applied these techniques in the development of highly scalable models to study biosocial and sociotechnical systems; this includes the transportation analysis and simulation system model for integrated urban transport planning [65] and models to study the spread of infectious disease in urban and national human populations, EpiSimdemics [58,66] and EpiFast [59], which are two very fast parallel codes.

Modeling Immune System using CGDDS

In ENISI, the immune system is represented using the CGDDS framework described above. The immune cells and bacteria represent the vertices (agents), and the phenotypes of the cells and bacteria represent the states. Cells can be located in four tissue sites: (i) lumen, (ii) epithelial barrier (EB), (iii) LP, and (iv) LN. If two cells are within a predefined spatial proximity, they are connected by an edge which represents a possible interaction between them. This interaction can change the state of the cell as defined by the state transition function. In general, there are three kinds of interactions: (i) interaction between a cell and a bacteria, (ii) interaction between two cells, and (iii) interaction between a cell and a group of cells.

To represent the state transition function, an appropriate automaton is used, which is defined for each cell type. Here, we use probabilistic timed transition systems (PTTS) to represent the automaton [58]. In PTTS, each state has an *id*, a set of attribute values, a dwell-time distribution, and one or more labeled sets of weighted transitions to other states. The label on the transition sets is used to select the appropriate set of transitions. The attributes of a state describe the features possessed by a cell that is in that state. Once a cell enters a state, the amount of time that it will remain in that state is drawn from the dwell-time distribution.

An illustrative description of this state chart-like formalism is given in Figure 6.1. In these depictions, arrows labeled with "i" indicate transitions that represent events in the inflammatory pathway and arrows labeled with "r" indicate transitions that represent those of the regulatory pathway. Ovals represent states of the automaton. Solid arrows represent time-dependent transitions labeled with the time in one state before transitioning to another. The dashed arrows represent single contact-dependent transitions, labeled with the set of interactor states necessary to induce state transition, and, in parenthesis, the probability of transition upon interaction. The default probability is 1. Dotted arrows represent multicontact dependent state transitions and are labeled with the function that determines the probability of interaction. Unlabeled solid arrows indicate that transition automatically occurs at the next update.

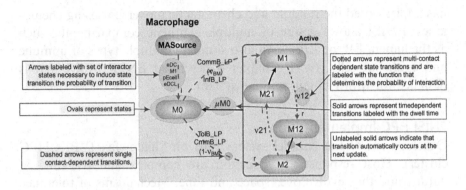

Figure 6.1 State chart-like description of a macrophage.

The contact dependency of state transitions in the graphical framework, as well as the need for computational efficiency, requires a number of approximations to the biological model. The CGDDS model stipulates that for a state change in one individual to be induced by another individual, the individuals must be colocated. Hence, the model cannot explicitly include induction of state transitions across location barriers as may occur when chemokines secreted by a cell in the LP influence migration of cells in the blood. To reduce complexity, individuals are not newly created or removed from the contact network G following the start of the simulation. Rather, biological processes that require these functions are either not included or represented in an indirect fashion. For example, the model does not include the constitutive flow of resting immune cells in and out of tissue or bacterial replication process.

AGENT-BASED MODELING USING ENISI

As shown in Refs. [1,2], ENISI can scale up to 576 processing elements (PEs) when simulating a population of 10^7 cells. Building on our previous work, ENISI MSM [67,68] integrates COPASI, the ODE solver, ENISI, the agent-based simulator and ValueLayer library from Repast, and the PDE solver to model cytokine and chemokine diffusion. COPASI [69], an ODE-based modeling tool, is widely used in computational biology for modeling "inside the cell." ENISI Visual [70] is an ABM tool built upon Repast Symphony, an open-source agent-based modeling and simulation platform, for simulating tissue-level immune responses and cell populations in the gut. ENISI Visual has implemented the random and chemotactic movement using chemokines. ENISI allows design of multiple synthetic compartments, such as the lumen, EB, or *LP*; it can also simulate multiple types of immune and epithelial cells (ECs). Chapter 8 described ENISI MSM that is designed for MSM of gut immune system.

ENISI HPC Implementation

Development of the parallel system runs on Shadowfax (VBI's HPC cluster). Host responses to infection are complex and dynamic in nature, and they evolve over space and time. Mechanisms of tolerance are modeled using graph theory principles designed specifically for dynamic systems. We are implementing and extending a CGDDS that was first introduced in computational epidemiology [71]. We have demonstrated in our previous models of enteric infection [1,55] that CGDDS is an intuitive and natural representation for the complex dynamical system that evolves over time and space. In addition, CGDDS can be efficiently parallelized to allow simulations of a significantly higher number of agents. ENISI HPC is written in C++ and utilizes the message passing interface (MPI) for interprocess communication. We have run ENISI HPC on a medium-sized cluster of 48 computing nodes, where each node consists of two 8-core Intel Sandy Bridge processors with 64 GB of RAM. ENISI HPC scales very well with large input size up to 10^7 cells. As our previous work [1,2] have shown, scaling the system beyond 10 million interactions requires significant programming effort to design efficient interprocess communication to effectively overlay communication with computation, effectively hiding communication latencies. Moreover, good load balancing and data locality remain hard programming challenges. Charm++ [72,73] is a task-driven parallel programming framework, where object-oriented (OO) principles can be used to write efficient HPC software. Charm++ provides built-in load balancing and communication optimization frameworks to enhance performance.

In Charm++, we represent each independent agent as a chare object. Similarly, each location patch is also represented as a chare object. A chare object can store data related to the agent or location. Chare objects for immune cells store information related to the cells, such as phenotypic information and intracellular models. The location chare objects store information, such as chemokine concentration, cytokine concentration, and cell types that reside in the location.

Like in immunological systems and host responses to pathogens, these chare objects can communicate with each other with message passing for computing diffusion with PDEs, performing intracellular model computation, and determining cellular movements. To achieve efficient parallelization, these chare objects are distributed among the processors. By combining VBI's modeling and data analytics capabilities, we will study tolerant host responses to pathogens across four scales of spatiotemporal magnitude as an information processing representation of mechanisms of protection against infection.

Immune systems have a number of important features that need to be captured by the above formalism. This leads to important changes and enhancements to the EpiSimdemics modeling environment on which ENISI is based. First, unlike EpiSimdemics, where the population was assumed to be a constant (deaths were simply captured by a vertex going to a specific state), ENISI requires that new cells are created as a result of interaction. This proliferation is an important aspect of an immune system. In fact, this modeling strategy captures the fact that creation of a new cell is context dependent. Thus, the above definition needs to be modified wherein the vertex state is not a constant. To keep the notation simple, this is not explicitly discussed above. Second, cells of one type, over the course of their lifecycle, become cells of another type. This phenotypic change is another important and novel aspect of such systems. In other words, the set of local functions and states associated with a node are not static. A natural way is to classify cells as having types (classes), each class has a set of states and specific kinds of interaction functions.

Finally, certain interactions are best represented as mentioned above as mean field interaction (e.g., concentration of cytokines). This is a modeling decision in a sense; we believe that this approximation preserves the basic features of the system, and the resulting dynamics will not be adversely affected by this representation.

ABM of *H. pylori*

Inflammatory bowel disease (IBD) is an immune-inflammatory condition of the gut, and it is initiated by an immune response to bacteria in the microflora, which results in lesions of the epithelial lining and LP. For further in depth details, refer Chapter 3. In the current biological model of IBD, a low-level inflammatory response is able to mount, from an initially small population, to a much larger population that is able to override the suppressive activity of its regulatory antagonists. Thus, an area of key interest to IBD intervention is identification of the specific interactions of the inflammatory pathways. An ODE-based model with 29 equations has been developed to describe the movement, interaction, and activation of inflammatory regulatory macrophages, T cells, and dendritic cells in the presence of bacteria and cytokines in the lumen, LP, and lymphoid tissue regions of gut mucosa [53]. Furthermore, *in silico* studies have been performed to trace the dynamics of inflammation markers back to specific interactions. Using an agent-based modeling approach [1], it was possible to simulate dysentery resulting from *Brachyispira hyodysenteriae* infection and identify aspects of the host immune pathways that lead to continued inflammation-induced tissue damage even after pathogen elimination. ENISI is a simulator of gastrointestinal immune mechanisms in response to resident commensal bacteria as well as invading pathogens. ENISI was used for the development of the ABMs. During the development of ENISI, three versions were released: ENISE HPC [1], ENISI Visual [70], and ENISI MSM [67]. ENISI HPC focuses on scalability by implementing a parallel simulation framework, ENISI visual focuses on visualizations, and ENISI MSM on the integration of heterogeneous modeling technologies for MSM purposes. ENISI MSM is further described in Chapter 8.

Mucosal immune response is well suited for an agent-based modeling approach because of its complexity, unique properties, and the types of available data. In addition, rule-based methods can be used to describe many of the events that take place during an inflammatory immune response (see Figure 6.1). For instance, the following behaviors can be formalized as rules in an ABM:

The inflammatory regulatory pathway:

1. A pathogen enters the lumen and contacts the EB.
2. Intestinal ECs switch to a pro-inflammatory phenotype (pEC) either in response to damage caused by the pathogen or by simple recognition of the pathogen. The pEC secretes microbicides and various signaling chemicals including cytokines and chemokines; it may also become permeable thus allowing pathogen entry into the LP [74]. Furthermore, immature dendritic cells in the lumen (iDCLumen) can internalize the pathogen and mature to be of effector phenotype

(eDC); these eDC can then migrate into the LP and present antigens (components of the pathogen) on their surfaces.

3. Chemicals secreted by damaged EC and eDC recruit resting macrophages (M0) and dendritic cells (iDC).
4. These macrophages and dendritic cells may contact and internalize the invading pathogen, which can lead to maturation of iDC to an effector phenotype and differentiation of macrophages to an inflammatory phenotype (M1).
5. Mature, antigen-presenting eDC recruits resting CD4+ T cells (resting T) to the LP and secrete cytokines that induce T cell differentiation to a pro-inflammatory Th1 or Th17 phenotype upon antigen recognition [75]. These stimulated T cells enter a transient state of proliferation (reproducing approximately 500 daughter cells of the same phenotype).
6. Presenting eDC to migrate to the LN and to contact resting memory and naive T cells by stimulating them to a Th1 or Th17 phenotype. The inflammatory T cells mature before migrating to the LP to be part of the inflammatory response at the site of infection.
7. At the infection site in the LP, Th1/Th17 cells secrete cytotoxins and cytokines that enhance secretion of inflammatory factors by surrounding T cells as well as induce additional macrophages to an M1 phenotype and T cells to a Th17 phenotype.
8. The EC damaged by factors derived from Th1, Th17, and M1 respond by secreting additional inflammatory cytokines resulting in openings in the EB, thus allowing direct pathogen entry into the LP. Finally, inflammation dissipates when pathogen is eliminated and direct immune cell stimulation ceases.

The anti-inflammatory regulatory pathway:

9. Upon internalization of the commensal or self-antigen, DCs differentiate to a tolerogenic phenotype (tDC) and macrophages differentiate to an M2 phenotype.
10. The tDC migrates to the LN where it becomes in contact and stimulates T cells to an iTreg phenotype. The latter move to the site of infection site in the LP.
11. M2 and tDC secrete anti-inflammatory cytokines (such as IL-10). The latter reduces inflammatory cytokine and cytotoxin production in surrounding immune cells. They also inducing the differentiation of T cells to T-regulatory cells (iTreg).
12. iTreg secrete additional IL-10; this increase induces differentiation of macrophages of the inflammatory phenotype to the regulatory

phenotype ($M1 \rightarrow M2$) and T cells of the Th17 phenotype to the iTreg phenotype [76]. These chances further promote the production of IL-10 and stimulation of T cells to iTreg.

13. Finally, an additional regulatory pathway involves natural T-regulatory cells (nTreg). These may have a reduced proliferation capacity compared to conventional T cells. Similar to the iTreg, nTreg secretes IL-10 promoting further M2 creation. Furthermore, nTreg binds eDC and inhibits their recruitment and stimulation of resting T cells to inflammatory phenotypes [77]. Certain genetic predispositions or immune dysfunctions can result in an inflammatory pathway being initiated by commensal bacteria strains [78]. (Figure 6.2).

As this example demonstrates, ABM approach can be very suitable for modeling the immune response process. As demonstrated, the system is complex but the number of interacting entities is limited. Each entity can have multiple phenotype (or states); individual-based behavior is important, and the spatiotemporal properties of the various

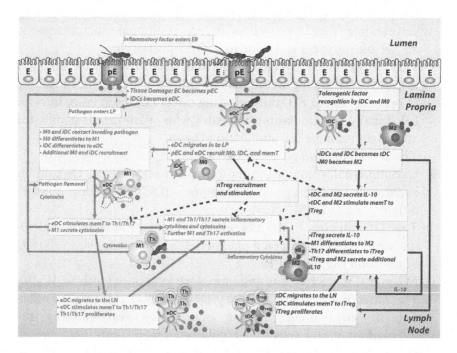

Figure 6.2 Events in the inflammatory (arrows labeled "i") and regulatory (arrows labeled "r") pathways. Dashed lines indicate inhibitory events.

entities can be a dominant factor in defining the overall system behavior. Finally, interaction between individual entities can be described by a set of rules; however, because of the complexity of the system, the overall system dynamics cannot be predicted without sufficient *in silico* simulations.

CALIBRATION AND VALIDATION OF THE PRELIMINARY MODEL

Simulations based on the model will provide population levels of all cell types, commensal and pathogenic bacteria, and cytokines over time in each tissue site.

Parameter values for a healthy individual are gathered from literature where possible, using pig, mouse, and human data. Unknown parameters are estimated by first estimating a range based on expert knowledge. From this range, the model will be calibrated to fit specific criteria for gut homeostasis in the absence of foreign bacteria at steady state. The criteria included the following: (i) T cell numbers reflect those measured in lymphoid tissue of healthy individuals. Specifically, in the LN concentrations of naive T cells and memory T cells are approximately 1.2×10^8/mL [57] and dendritic cells are 10^6/mL [79], (ii) no commensal bacteria is seen in the LP, but lumen population upholds an active immune cell population with tolerogenic mediators detected, (iii) the lumen bacteria stays within a concentration of $10^{11}-10^{12}$/ml [80], (iv) the EC layer remains unchanged with an average concentration of 10^4 individuals per milliliter [80], (v) active and resting nTreg compose approximately 10% of the total CD4+ T cell population [81], (vi) the level of deactivating cytokine-secreting cells in the LP are significantly higher than activating cytokine-secreting cell levels [82], and (vii) a single DC contacts up to 500 T cells/hour in the LN [83].

The model was validated by adding pathogenic bacteria to the system at time point 0 in the lumen at a dose of concentration of 10^8 cells and observing the same qualitative population dynamics as those in animal studies [84,85]. Specifically, that (i) the most significant cell population increase is among effector phenotypes, (ii) inflammation coincides with a depletion of the EC layer, (iii) immunity and EC depletion coincide with an increased rate of bacterial migration across the EB and accumulation in the LP, (iv) immunity coincides with an increased rate of M2 macrophages switching to M1, and (v) recovery is observed coinciding with reversion of all macrophages back to M2, return of the EC concentration to the basal level, reduction of inflammatory cell types to homeostatic levels, and elimination of bacteria from the LP.

SENSITIVITY ANALYSIS FOR ABM

Sensitivity analysis for the ABM is to study how the variation in the output of a system can be apportioned to different input parameters [86]. In other words, sensitivity analysis tries to determine how the change of input parameters would affect the change of the output. There are many applications of sensitivity analysis to exploit the inherent knowledge of data, to quantify the uncertainty of the system, to optimize the design of a system, and to rank the influence of various parameters on the system [87]. Thus, sensitivity analysis for ABMs can provide a comprehensive understanding of the influence of the different input parameters and their variations on the model outcomes.

There are generally two types of sensitivity analysis for a complex ABM: global sensitivity analysis and local sensitivity analysis. Both statistical and deterministic methods are used for sensitivity analysis for the purpose of the study. Global sensitivity analysis aims to evaluate the entire parameter space to determine the system's functionality [87,88]. It would help gain an overall vision of the system, especially useful for distinguishing significant parameter from the insignificant input parameters. Common approaches for global sensitivity analysis include variance decomposition, response surface methodologies [89,90] and surrogate modeling approach [91,92]. Based on the global sensitivity analysis, one can often focus the effort on certain parameters or regions of particular interest, which is referred as the local sensitivity analysis. That is, the local sensitivity analysis is to analyze the effects of local changes of a parameter in the system [93]. It can further gain more insight of the system for the local structure of the system. Typical methodology for the local sensitivity analysis is one-factor-at-a-time [94].

The choice of the specific method for sensitivity analysis is determined based on the inherent characteristics of the system under study.

It is worth noting that complex systems with expensive computation cost could limit the scope of sensitivity analysis to some extent. For the ABM such as ENISI, the objective of the sensitivity analysis is to identify the most significant parameters in the model and to quantify how the parameter uncertainty influences the outcomes. For a complex ABM, it is very challenging to analytically explore the behavior of the system due to the large number of parameters [90]. To effectively conduct sensitivity analysis, the ABM needs to be evaluated with different values of the input parameters under a specified number of runs. To address this challenge, an efficient design of experiments is very important. For the sensitivity analysis of ABM, we adopt an experimental design strategy [94–96] using orthogonal arrays (OAs) to obtain a sparse design with desirable properties. Designs of OA [97] have been widely used in many engineering applications. Specifically, an OA with strength t experimental design is a design matrix such that for every t columns, the possible distinct rows appear the same number of times. Such a property maintains a good balance of level assignment for each factor.

Based on the results of sensitivity analysis, a reduced model with a smaller set of significant parameters can be produced. Sensitivity analysis is important for understanding relationship between input parameters and outputs, testing the robustness of the output, quantifying uncertainty, and identifying optimal parameter settings in the model. The goals of sensitivity analysis in ABM include (1) evaluating the influence of parameters, (2) ranking the significance of parameters based on their influence, and (3) quantifying uncertainty of the model.

Influence of Parameters

Each parameter in the ABM can have different levels of values. From the outputs, we can observe different patterns of behaviors of parameters with the change of levels. For some parameters with the increase or decrease on the level of the parameter value, the quantity of interest in the output can also increases or decreases, which is called monotonic effect. A different pattern for some parameters can also occur, where with the increase (or decrease) of parameter value, the output increases (or decreases) to a maximum (or minimum) peak, then starts decreasing (or increasing) again. There can also have an interesting pattern, which expresses a drastic change between two parameter levels, but not much change observed between the other consecutive parameter levels. Those patterns reflect different mechanisms how input parameters affect the output of the systems.

Ranking of Parameters

To determine the level of impact of parameters on the ABM, a first attempt is the analysis of variance (ANOVA) to find the significant parameters. Specifically, the response for the ANOVA is obtained from quantity of interest in the output. By applying the ANOVA considering the main effects model, the observed variance in the output response is partitioned into components attributable to different parameters. Consequently, the ANOVA provides a statistical test of whether or not each parameter plays a significant role to contribute the observed total variation of output responses. A statistically significant result with p value less than a threshold (significance level) justifies the rejection of the null hypothesis that the parameter is insignificant. It provides an efficient technique to determine the sensitivity of each parameter with respect to the output. Then, the top sensitive parameters can be selected based on their p values. This set of most sensitive parameters is used to fine tune the parameters of models.

Quantifying Uncertainty

To quantify the complex relations between inputs and output, uncertainty quantification with surrogate models (e.g., Gaussian process modeling) are often used for computer simulations [91,98]. In the application of ABM such as ENISI, the number of input variables can be large, and there can be multiple responses in the output. Multivariate Gaussian process can be a good candidate model as emulator for uncertainty quantification. It is also crucial to identify important parameters through the functional ANOVA based on the estimated model. Since the final estimated model is a predictive model from the computer simulations, it can provide a rigorous investigation with quantification of uncertainty with respect to parameters and response surface [99,100].

SCALING THE SENSITIVITY ANALYSIS CALCULATIONS

One key challenge for the sensitivity analysis of ABM lies in the size and number of parameters of the model and the computational cost associated with the stochastic nature of the process. A simulation in ABM such as ENISI consists of a magnitude of individual agents.

Specifically, there are 30 different types of agents and a few hundred individual rules. On a modern HPC cluster of 48 nodes, a single run of the simulation takes about 90 min on average. Because of this limitation, the runtime of multiple simulations must be taken into consideration. For conducting sensitivity analysis at such an intensive computational scale, an efficient design of experiments is crucial for enabling the extraction of useful information and model-driven hypothesis generation.

The sensitivity analysis of ENISI represents an illustration example. There are 25 parameters considered to be continuous. However, if a parameter takes only four different values, then a full factorial experimental design would require $4^{25} = 1.126 \times 10^{15}$ runs, which is not possible in terms of the system's runtime. To alleviate this problem, one can use an OA with 128 runs, which is a more realistic number of simulation. Such a design makes each column mutually orthogonal to each other. Therefore, the variance-based model using such a design allows the estimated main effect uncorrelated with each other. This design has the following attractive properties: (i) projecting the design points onto any factor, there are exactly 16 replicates for each level; (ii) projecting the design points onto any two variables (i.e., any two columns of the design matrix), it is a full factorial (four-by-four) with eight replications for each level combination. The proposed design is sparse in the sense that there are only 128 points in a 25-dimensional space, while the design points are well spread out with good properties. Therefore, the proposed design enables the effective study of the main effect of any factor.

SCALABILITY AND PERFORMANCE

To understand the performance of ENISI HPC implementation, the system is evaluated against multiple problem sizes ranging from 10^5 to 10^7 cells. Each experiment has a time step of 250 simulation days. The HPC cluster used for the evaluation consists of total 62 compute nodes. Each node comprised two 6-core Intel Xeon X5670 processors and 48 GB of 1333 MHz DDR3 memory. The implementation used MVAPICH2 MPI over a Mellanox 40 Gb/s dual-port QDR InfiniBand interconnect.

Table 6.1 lists the data set sizes used and the fastest simulation execution time achieved for each of the data sets. Figure 6.3a plots the simulation execution time for different number of PEs for each of the

Table 6.1 Data Set Sizes and Simulation Execution Times for 250 Simulation Days

Problem Size	N_{cells}	Execution Time	N_{nodes}	N_{cores}	Message Coalescing Buffer Size	Memory Usage of PE_0 (MB)	Parallel Efficiency	Communication Overhead (%)
10^5	100,038	00:00:41	16	192	10	161	0.24	22.6
10^5	1,000,594	00:02:26	32	384	10	168	0.73	22.2
10^5	10,000,110	01:26:48	48	576	1000	340	0.94	6.5
10^5	100,001,314	226:39:10	56	672	1000	814	N/A	50.1

The execution time (hh:mm:ss) and number of nodes are given for the fastest running configuration for each problem size.

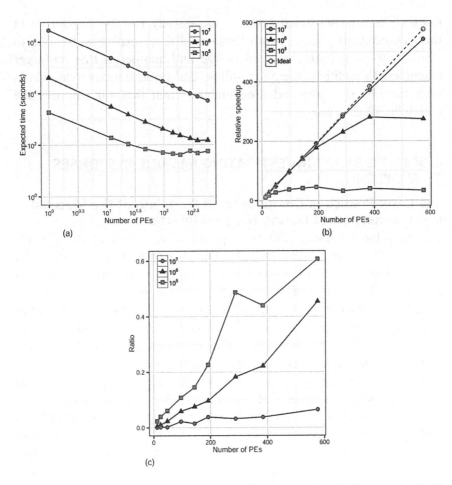

Figure 6.3 Scalability of ENteric Immunity SImulator on different sized problems. (a) Execution time for 250 iterations; (b) Speedup; (c) Ratio of communication to total execution time.

data sets used. Figure 6.3b shows the speedup achieved for each of the data sets. For the small-sized problem with 105 cells, the simulation scales only up to 192 PEs and gains a speedup of up to 45. However, for a medium size problem with 10^6 cells, the scalability extends to more PEs (up to 384 PEs), gaining a speedup of 280. For the largest size problem with 10^7 cells, it scales with all the 576 PEs that we used and achieves a speedup of up to 543, which is 94% of the ideal speedup, finishing in just 1.5 h. We believe that the 10^5 and 10^6 problem sizes have too little data at larger core counts, leading to poor parallel efficiency. For an extremely large problem with 10^8 cells, we were unable to evaluate the scaling on the test machine as the network resource became saturated but can successfully run the simulation at this unprecedented scale. From these results, we expect to be able to continue to scale both the problem size and number of PEs on larger machines. In addition, there are still several optimizations available in both the ENISI model and the simulator itself that will improve the scalability of the system.

MODELING STUDY INVESTIGATING IMMUNE RESPONSES TO *H. PYLORI*

Use Case: Predictive Computational Modeling of the Mucosal Immune Responses During *H. pylori* Infection

To study the mucosal immune response to *H. pylori* at the systems level locally in the gastric mucosa, ODE in combination with ABM was used [55]. The discussion below follows the results described in Ref. [46]. During the initial step of model development, ODE-based models were used to shed lights on the CD4+ T cell distribution after infection as well as the role of peroxisome proliferator-activated receptor γ (PPARγ) during infection. The parameters estimated through the ODE-based modeling were used as a starting point for the ABM step. Agent-based modeling added some randomness to the system and helped in the representation of complex cellular responses by also taking into consideration individual and emerging behavior of cells as well as their spatiotemporal features. The ABM was able to better represent the cross-link, complex, and nonlinear processes with multiple feedback loops. Furthermore, by incorporating spatiotemporal features in the model and integrating multiples scales in a unified way, the resulting model of the mucosal immune response to *H. pylori* was successful at predicting novel testable hypothesis. The computational model of *H. pylori* predicted a crucial contribution of Th1 and Th17 effector responses as mediators of histopathological changes in the gastric mucosa during chronic stages of infection. These hypotheses were experimentally validated in mice models.

We also investigate the potential role of PPARγ, a nuclear receptor and transcription factor whose activation has been observed to modulate host responses to *H. pylori* using loss-of-function approaches. In order to investigate the role of PPARγ in mucosal immune responses to *H. pylori in silico*, we also implemented T cell and myeloid cell-specific PPARγ knockout models. Specifically, to create an *in silico* cell-specific knockout model, rates of regulatory phenotype differentiation were lowered and rates controlling effector response in both LP and glutamine (GLN) were increased. Upon observing immune-pathogenesis *in silico*, we analyzed the contact network to identify specific mechanisms of pathogenicity. The results identified specific processes associated with the infection that do and do not contribute to this simulated pathogenesis. A comprehensive analysis of this model along with differential equation-based model is studied in Ref. [54].

H. pylori [101] was represented by assigning functions to commensal bacteria representing a combination of the immune-modulatory mechanisms mentioned. As default, it was assumed to have all possible effects on ECs. Specifically, infection was simulated *in silico* by adding commensal bacteria on day 2 and following the state changes and migration of cells over 60 days. The model was fit to qualitative trends observed among tissue samples of mice experimentally infected with *H. pylori* strain 26695, compared to the control group, gathered by collaborators. In these experiments, both LP and GLN tissue samples were taken from infected and control mice on days 7, 14, 30, and 60 postinfection, and the count of cells of each regulatory/inflammatory phenotype was determined through flow cytometry.

Figure 6.4 depicts the dynamics of T cell populations over the course of 60-day infections. Results show a significant increase in the concentration of CD4+ T cells in both the gastric LP and the GLN. Taking a closer look at CD4+ T cell subsets following infection in the wild-type model, we observed that in the GLN, Th1 cells peaked on day 30 postinfection and remained at high levels with fairly constant values throughout the rest of the infection period (Figure 6.4a,d). Th17 responses were induced in the GLN and later detected in the LP, together with a regulatory T cell response that persisted over time in both gastric LP (Figure 6.4b,c) and GLN (Figure 6.4e,f). The experimental data collected from *in vivo* experiments also validates the T cells outputs [55]. We observed that the rise in T cells occurs in conjunction with a rise is effector dendritic cell levels in the LP. This increase in immune activity is associated with mounting epithelial damage represented by transition of EC automata from the healthy cell state to the activated pro-EC state and from the activated pro-EC state to the dead cell state. To identify the pathways by which this mounting immune response is associated with tissue damage, we focus on one

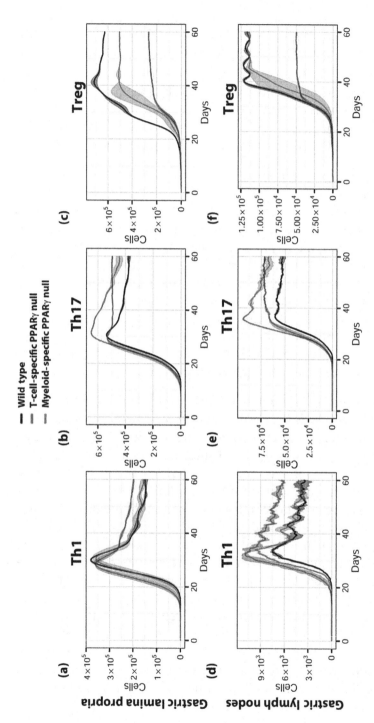

Figure 6.4 Dynamics of T-cell populations over a period of 60 days in the presence of H. pylori. (a–c) Number of Th1, Th17 and Treg cells in the Gastric lamina propria; (d–f) Number of Th1, Th17 and Treg cells in the Gastric lymph nodes.

specific simulation replicate that resulted in the greatest epithelial damage and identified the states of neighbors that induced key health state-defining state changes.

It was found that for all cells that underwent the transition healthy EC to activated pro-EC phenotype, the transition is primarily induced by *H. pylori* directly in the earlier stages of infection (days 1–30). However, in the chronic stage (days 30–60 postinfection), when the pro-inflammatory immune response is triggered in response to the pathogen, epithelial damage is occurring through contact with IFNγ-secreting Th1 cells, instead of being caused by the direct effects of the bacterium. Indeed, for all the cells that underwent the transition activated pro-EC to dead cell, this occurred only upon contact with neighbors in the Th1 state.

T cells may be stimulated by macrophages, dendritic cells in the LP, or "sampling" dendritic cells in the lumen. It was found that all individuals that stimulated T cells to a Th1 phenotype were in the effector "sampling" dendritic cell state, indicating "sampling" dendritic cells are solely responsible for T cell stimulation over the entire 60-day infection in this case. As the count of individuals in the effector "sampling" dendritic cell state remains relatively constant over the course of infection, the only explanation for the continued rise in Th1 is an increase in resting T cells in the LP that are being recruited to the infection site and subsequently stimulated. To identify which cells were responsible for this recruitment, Figure 6.5 depicts the number of individuals in each state that induce the recruitments of resting T cells. It can be observed that pro-inflammatory ECs, stimulated by *H. pylori* and Th1, which together with effector dendritic cells that are also stimulated by *H. pylori*, are equal contributors to resting T cell recruitment. This identifies a positive feedback loop that is fed by the *H. pylori* presence in which *H. pylori*-damaged EC secrete chemo-attractants that recruit resting T cells. These are subsequently stimulated to Th1, which contribute to further epithelial damage leading to increased chemoattractant secretion and T cell recruitment (Figure 6.5).

Although *H. pylori* appears to be contributing to epithelial damage and the parameter set maximizes its ability to degrade epithelial tight junctions, no individuals representing *H. pylori* are seen in the LP. This was explained by finding that the majority of commensal bacteria that changes to dead state, made the decision when in contact with

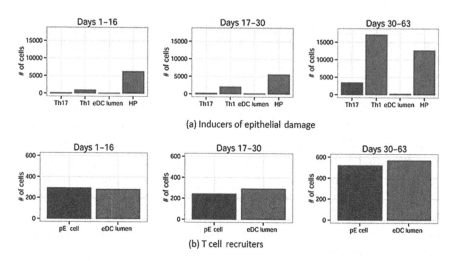

Figure 6.5 *Epithelial damage and T-cell recruitment. (a) The counts of individuals in each state that induce epithelial damage over simulated infection period. (b) The counts of individuals in each that recruit a T cell to the lamina propria during the course of the simulation infection.*

neighbors in the microbicide-secreting pro-EC state. This indicates that in this *in silico* scenario, although *H. pylori* is effective in degrading epithelial tight junctions, the fact that it also induces secretion of microbicides, such as defensin through the NF-κβ pathway, ensures the elimination prior to migration into the LP, thus canceling out any benefit that may come from this CagA + -encoded function.

CONCLUDING REMARKS

Among various models of immune pathways studied, ABM-based frameworks are unique in their representational capability and scalability. With proper formal representation, modeling, and careful implementation, ABM could be an extremely useful tool for study of immune systems. The framework is an important first step towards a system that will be useful for immunologists, bioinformaticians, and infectious disease experts in their everyday work. The next generation ENISI tool, known as ENISI MSM, has similar scalability and can perform across scales using ABM and ODE modeling as described in Chapter 8.

ACKNOWLEDGMENT

We thank our external collaborators and members of the Network Dynamics and Simulation Science Laboratory for their suggestions and comments. This work has been partially supported by DTRA Grant HDTRA1-11-1-0016, DTRA CNIMS Contract HDTRA1-11-D-0016-0001, NIH MIDAS Grant 2U01GM070694-09, NSF NetSe CNS-1011769. This work was also supported in part by National Institute of Allergy and Infectious Diseases Contract No. HHSN272201000056C to J. Bassaganya-Riera and funds from the Nutritional Immunology and Molecular Medicine Laboratory (www.nimml.org).

REFERENCES

[1] Wendelsdorf KV, et al. ENteric Immunity SImulator: a tool for in silico study of gastroenteric infections. IEEE Trans Nanobioscience 2012;11(3):273−88.

[2] Bisset K, et al. High-performance interaction-based simulation of gut immunopathologies with ENteric Immunity SImulator (ENISI). 2012 IEEE 26th International Parallel and Distributed Processing Symposium (IPDPS); 2012. p. 48−59.

[3] Wendelsdorf KV, et al. ENteric Immunity Simulator: a tool for *in silico* study of gut immunopathologies. Proceedings of the IEEE International Conference Bioinformatics and Biomedicine; 2011.

[4] Epstein JM, Cummings DAT, Chakravarty S, Singa RM, Burke DS. Toward a containment strategy for smallpox bioterror: an individual-based computational approach. Complexity 2002;4157 Press.

[5] Macal C, North M. Tutorial on agent-based modeling and simulation. J Simul 2010;8 (2):177−83.

[6] Parunak HV, Savit R, Riolo RL. Agent-based modeling vs. equation-based modeling: a case study and users' guide. Multi Agent Syst Agent-Based Simulation 1998;1534:10−25.

[7] Materi W, Wishart DS. Computational systems biology in drug discovery and development: methods and applications. Drug Discov Today 2007;12(7−8):295−303.

[8] Arciero JC, et al. Using a mathematical model to analyze the role of probiotics and inflammation in necrotizing enterocolitis. PLoS One 2010;5(4):e10066.

[9] Wigginton JE, Kirschner D. A model to predict cell-mediated immune regulatory mechanisms during human infection with Mycobacterium tuberculosis. J Immunol 2001;166 (3):1951−67.

[10] Blaser MJ, Kirschner D. The equilibria that allow bacterial persistence in human hosts. Nature 2007;449(7164):843−9.

[11] Blaser MJ, Kirschner D. Dynamics of Helicobacter pylori colonization in relation to the host response. Proc Natl Acad Sci USA 1999;96(15):8359−64.

[12] Perelson AS. Modelling viral and immune system dynamics. Nat Rev Immunol 2002;2 (1):28−36.

[13] Antia R, et al. Models of CD8 + responses: 1. What is the antigen-independent proliferation program. J Theor Biol 2003;221(4):585−98.

[14] Carneiro J, et al. Immunological self-tolerance: lessons from mathematical modeling. J Comput Appl Math 2005;184:77−100.

[15] Wodarz D, Thomsen AR. Effect of the CTL proliferation program on virus dynamics. Int Immunol 2005;17(9):1269−76.

[16] Shahaf G, Johnson K, Mehr R. B cell development in aging mice: lessons from mathematical modeling. Int Immunol 2006;18(1):31−9.

[17] Kim PS, Lee PP, Levy D. Modeling regulation mechanisms in the immune system. J Theor Biol 2007;246(1):33−69.

[18] Colijn C, Mackey MC. A mathematical model of hematopoiesis: II. Cyclical neutropenia. J Theor Biol 2005;237(2):133−46.

[19] Onsum M, Rao CV. A mathematical model for neutrophil gradient sensing and polarization. PLoS Comput Biol 2007;3(3):e36.

[20] Figge MT. Optimization of immunoglobulin substitution therapy by a stochastic immune response model. PLoS One 2009;4(5):e5685.

[21] Bonabeau E, Dorigo M, Theraulaz G. Swarm intelligence: from natural to artificial systems. New York: Oxford University Press, Inc; 1999.

[22] Dong X, et al. Agent-based modeling of endotoxin-induced acute inflammatory response in human blood leukocytes. PLoS One 2010;5(2):e9249.

[23] Forrest S, Beauchemin C. Computer immunology. Immunol Rev 2007;216(1):176−97.

[24] Bauer AL, Beauchemin CAA, Perelson AS. Agent-based modeling of host-pathogen systems: the successes and challenges. Inf Sci 2009;179(10):1379−89.

[25] Fachada N, Lopes VV, Rosa A. Agent based modelling and simulation of the immune system: a review. Lisboa, Portugal: Systems and Robotics Institute, Instituto Superior Tecnico; 2000.

[26] An G. Introduction of an agent-based multi-scale modular architecture for dynamic knowledge representation of acute inflammation. Theor Biol Med Model 2008;5:11.

[27] Vodovotz Y, et al. *In silico* models of acute inflammation in animals. Shock 2006;26 (3):235−44.

[28] Baldazzi V, Castiglione F, Bernaschi M. An enhanced agent based model of the immune system response. Cell Immunol 2006;244:77−9.

[29] Mi Q, et al. Agent-based model of inflammation and wound healing: insights into diabetic foot ulcer pathology and the role of transforming growth factor-β1. Wound Repair Regen 2007;15:671−82.

[30] An G. Agent-based computer simulation and sirs: building a bridge between basic science and clinical trials. Shock 2001;16:266−73.

[31] Grilo A, Caetano A, Rosa A. Agent-based artificial immune system. In: 2001 Genetic and evolutionary computation conference late breaking papers; 2001.

[32] Tay JC, Jhavar A. CAFISS: a complex adaptive framework for immune system simulation. In: Proceedings of the 2005 ACM symposium on applied computing. ACM: Santa Fe, New Mexico; 2005. p. 158−64.

[33] Celada F, Seiden PE. A computer model of cellular interactions in the immune system. Immunol Today 1992;13(2):56−62.

[34] Castiglione F, et al. Simulating Epstein−Barr virus infection with C-ImmSim. Bioinformatics 2007;23:1371−7.

[35] Bernaschi M, Castiglione F. Design and implementation of an immune system simulator. Comput Biol Med 2001;31(5):303−31.

[36] Emerson A, Rossi E. ImmunoGrid: the virtual human immune system project. Stud Health Technol Inform 2007:56−62.

[37] Efroni S, Harel D, Cohen IR. Reactive animation: realistic modeling of complex dynamic systems. Computer 2005:38−47.

[38] Swerdlin N, Cohen IR, Harel D. The lymph node B cell immune response: dynamic analysis *in-silico*. Proc IEEE 2008;96(8):1421−43.

[39] Mata J, Cohn M. Cellular automata-based modeling program: synthetic immune system. Immunol Rev 2007;216(1):198−212.

[40] Meier-Schellersheim M, Mack G. SIMMUNE, a tool for simulating and analyzing immune system behavior. CoRR; 1999. cs.MA/9903017.

[41] Sneddon MW, Faeder JR, Emonet T. Efficient modeling, simulation and coarse-graining of biological complexity with NFsim. Nat Methods 2011;8(2):177–83.

[42] Folcik VA, An GC, Orosz CG. The Basic Immune Simulator: an agent-based model to study the interactions between innate and adaptive immunity. Theor Biol Med Model 2007;4:39.

[43] Sutterlin T, et al. Modeling multi-cellular behavior in epidermal tissue homeostasis via finite state machines in multi-agent systems. Bioinformatics 2009;25(16):2057–63.

[44] Pappalardo F, et al. Computational simulations of the immune system for personalized medicine: state of the art and challenges. System 2008:1–36.

[45] North MJ, et al. Complex adaptive systems modeling with Repast Simphony. Complex Adaptive Syst Model 2013;1:3.

[46] Collier N, Howe TR, North MJ. Onward and upward: the transition to Repast 2.0. Proceedings of the first annual North American Association for Computational Social and Organizational Science conference. Pittsburgh: Carnegie Mellon University; 2003.

[47] Sallach D, Macal C. Introduction: the simulation of social agents Special Issue Soc Sci Comput Rev 2001;19(3):245–8.

[48] Kim PS, Lee PP. Modeling protective anti-tumor immunity via preventative cancer vaccines using a hybrid agent-based and delay differential equation approach. PLoS Comput Biol 2012;8(10):e1002742.

[49] Marino S, El-Kebir M, Kirschner D. A hybrid multi-compartment model of granuloma formation and T cell priming in tuberculosis. J Theor Biol 2011;280(1):50–62.

[50] An G. A model of TLR4 signaling and tolerance using a qualitative, particle-event-based method: introduction of spatially configured stochastic reaction chambers (SCSRC). Math Biosci 2009;217(1):43–52.

[51] Angermann BR, et al. Computational modeling of cellular signaling processes embedded into dynamic spatial contexts. Nat Methods 2012;9(3):283–9.

[52] Meier-Schellersheim M, et al. Key role of local regulation in chemosensing revealed by a new molecular interaction-based modeling method. PLoS Comput Biol 2006;2(7):e82.

[53] Wendelsdorf K, et al. Model of colonic inflammation: immune modulatory mechanisms in inflammatory bowel disease. J Theor Biol 2010;264(4):1225–39.

[54] Carbo A, et al. Systems modeling of molecular mechanisms controlling cytokine-driven CD4+ T cell differentiation and phenotype plasticity. PLoS Comput Biol 2013;9(4): e1003027.

[55] Carbo A, et al. Predictive computational modeling of the mucosal immune responses during *Helicobacter pylori* infection. PLoS One 2013;8(9):e73365.

[56] Beauchemin CAA. Agent-based models in infectious disease and immunology. Springer Encyclopedia Appl Comput Math. Springer-Verlag, Germany 2012.

[57] Haase AT. Population biology of HIV-1 infection: viral and CD4+ T cell demographics and dynamics in lymphatic tissues. Annu Rev Immunol 1999;17:625–56.

[58] Barrett C, Bisset K, Eubank S, Feng X, Marathe M. EpiSimdemics: an efficient algorithm for simulating the spread of infectious disease over large realistic social networks. In: SuperComputing 08 INternational conference for high performance computing, networking, storage, and analysis. Austin, TX; 2008.

[59] Eubank S, et al. Modelling disease outbreaks in realistic urban social networks. Nature 2004;429(6988):180–4.

[60] Halloran ME, et al. Modeling targeted layered containment of an influenza pandemic in the United States. Proc Natl Acad Sci USA 2008;105(12):4639–44.

[61] Mortveit HS, Reidys CM. Universitext An introduction to sequential dynamical systems. Springer; 2008. vol. I–XII, p. 1248.

[62] Barrett C, Beckman R, Berkbigler K, Bisset K, Bush B, Campbell K, et al., TRANSIMS: Transportation analysis simulation system, 2001 Los Alamos National Laboratory Unclassfied Report, Tech. Rep. LA-UR-00-1725.

[63] Barrett E, et al. Rapid screening method for analyzing the conjugated linoleic acid production capabilities of bacterial cultures. Appl Environ Microbiol 2007;73:2333–7.

[64] Karaoz U, et al. Whole-genome annotation by using evidence integration in functional-linkage networks. Proceedings of the National Academy of Sciences of the United States of America; 2004.

[65] Ohta T, et al. An intelligent search engine and GUI-based efficient MEDLINE search tool based on deep syntactic parsing. Proceedings of the COLING/ACL on interactive presentation sessions. Morristown, NJ: Association for Computational Linguistics; 2006. p. 17–20.

[66] Yeom J-S, et al. Overcoming the scalability challenges of epidemic simulations on blue waters. IEEE 28th International Parallel and Distributed Processing Symposium; 2014.

[67] Mei Y, et al. ENISI MSM: a novel multi-scale modeling platform for computational immunology. In: 2014 IEEE International Conference on Bioinformatics and Biomedicine. Belfast, UK; 2014. p. 391–96.

[68] Mei Y, Abedi V, Carbo A, Zhang X, Lu P, Philipson C, et al. Multiscale modeling of mucosal immune responses. BMC Bioinformatics 2015;16(Suppl. 12):S2.

[69] Hoops S, et al. COPASI—a COmplex PAthway SImulator. Bioinformatics 2006;22 (24):3067–74.

[70] Mei Y, et al. ENISI Visual, an agent-based simulator for modeling gut immunity. IEEE International Conference of Bioinformatics and Biomedicine (BIBM); 2012.

[71] Barrett CL, et al. Interactions among human behavior, social networks, and societal infrastructures: a case study in computational epidemiology. In: Ravi SS, Shukla SK, editors. Fundamental problems in computing. Netherlands: Springer Science; 2009. p. 477–507.

[72] Kale LV, Zheng G. Charm++: parallel programming with message-driven objects. In: Wilson GV, Paul, Lu P, editors. Parallel programming using C++. Cambridge, MA: MIT Press; 1996.

[73] Bisset KR, et al. Contagion diffusion with EpiSimdemics. In: Kale LV, Bhatele A, editors. Parallel science and engineering applications: the charm++ approach. Taylor & Francis Group, CRC Press; 2014.

[74] Hill DA, Artis D. Intestinal bacteria and the regulation of immune cell homeostasis. Annu Rev Immunol 2010;28:623–67.

[75] Iwasaki A. Mucosal dendritic cells. Annu Rev Immunol 2007;25:381–418.

[76] Gordon S, Taylor PR. Monocyte and macrophage heterogeneity. Nat Rev Immunol 2005;5 (12):953–64.

[77] Onishi Y, et al. Foxp3 + natural regulatory T cells preferentially form aggregates on dendritic cells in vitro and actively inhibit their maturation. Proc Natl Acad Sci USA 2008;105 (29):10113–18.

[78] Ng SC, et al. Intestinal dendritic cells: their role in bacterial recognition, lymphocyte homing, and intestinal inflammation. Inflamm Bowel Dis 2010;16(10):1787–807.

[79] Catron DM, et al. Visualizing the first 50 hr of the primary immune response to a soluble antigen. Immunity 2004;21(3):341–7.

[80] Artis D. Epithelial-cell recognition of commensal bacteria and maintenance of immune homeostasis in the gut. Nat Rev Immunol 2008;8(6):411−20.

[81] Asano M, et al. Autoimmune disease as a consequence of developmental abnormality of a T cell subpopulation. J Exp Med 1996;184(2):387−96.

[82] Uhlig HH, et al. Characterization of Foxp3(+)CD4(+)CD25(+) and IL-10-secreting CD4(+) CD25(+) T cells during cure of colitis. J Immunol 2006;177(9):5852−60.

[83] von Andrian UH, Mempel TR. Homing and cellular traffic in lymph nodes. Nat Rev Immunol 2003;3(11):867−78.

[84] Hontecillas R, et al. CD4+ T-cell responses and distribution at the colonic mucosa during Brachyspira hyodysenteriae-induced colitis in pigs. Immunology 2005;115(1):127−35.

[85] Jonasson R, et al. Immunological alterations during the clinical and recovery phases of experimental swine dysentery. J Med Microbiol 2006;55(Pt 7):845−55.

[86] Saltelli A, Chan K, Scott EM. Sensitivity analysis. Wiley series in probability and statistics. Chichester; New York: Wiley; 2000. vol. xv, 475 p.

[87] Cacuci DG, Ionescu-Bujor M, Navon IM. Sensitivity and uncertainty analysis. Boca Raton: Chapman & Hall/CRC Press; 2003. vol. v, <1-2>

[88] Hamby DM. A comparison of sensitivity analysis techniques. Health Phys 1995;68 (2):195−204.

[89] Saltelli A, et al. Sensitivity analysis in practice: a guide to assessing scientific models. New York, NY: Halsted Press; 2004.

[90] Helton JC. Uncertainty and sensitivity analysis for models of complex systems. Computational methods in transport: verification and validation. Berlin, Heidelberg: Springer; 2008. p. 207−28.

[91] Sacks J, et al. Design and analysis of computer experiments. Stat Sci 1989:409−23.

[92] Santner TJ, Williams BJ, Notz W. The design and analysis of computer experiments. Springer series in statistics. New York: Springer; 2003. vol. xii, 283 p.

[93] Frey HC, Patil SR. Identification and review of sensitivity analysis methods. Risk Anal 2002;22(3):553−78.

[94] Lee HY, et al. Simulation and prediction of the adaptive immune response to influenza a virus infection. J Virol 2009;83(14):7151−65.

[95] Box GE, Hunter JS, Hunter WG. Statistics for experimenters: design, innovation, and discovery. AMC 2005;10:12.

[96] Montgomery DC. Design and analysis of experiments. Cary, North Carolina, USA: SAS Institute Inc; 2012.

[97] Hedayat AS, Sloane NJA, Stufken J. Orthogonal arrays: theory and applications. New York: Springer-Verlag; 1999.

[98] Cressie N. Statistics for spatial data. Terra Nova 1992;4(5):613−17.

[99] Kennedy MC, O'Hagan A. Bayesian calibration of computer models. J R Stat Soc Ser B Stat Methodol 2001;63:425−50.

[100] Bayarri MJ, et al. A framework for validation of computer models. Technometrics 2007;49 (2):138−54.

[101] Mane SP, et al. Host-interactive genes in Amerindian *Helicobacter pylori* diverge from their old world homologs and mediate inflammatory responses. J Bacteriol 2010;192 (12):3078−92.

CHAPTER 7

From Big Data Analytics and Network Inference to Systems Modeling

Pawel Michalak[1], Bruno W. Sobral[2], Vida Abedi[1], Young Bun Kim[1], Xinwei Deng[3], Casandra Philipson[4], Monica Viladomiu[1], Pinyi Lu[1], Katherine Wendelsdorf[5], Raquel Hontecillas[1], and Josep Bassaganya-Riera[1]

[1]Nutritional Immunology and Molecular Medicine Laboratory, Virginia Bioinformatics Institute, Virginia Tech, Blacksburg, VA, USA [2]One Health Institute, Colorado State University, Fort Collins, CO, USA [3]Department of Statistics, Virginia Tech, Blacksburg, VA, USA [4]Biotherapeutics Inc., Blacksburg, VA, USA [5]Applied Advanced Genomics, QIAGEN, Redwood City, CA, USA

INTRODUCTION

In silico experimentation is a very powerful tool for model-driven hypothesis generation and could significantly improve design of pre-clincal and clinical studies. However, predictive computational modeling requires sufficient data for the learning process and model calibration. These data-rich models that are well calibrated with experimental data can be then used to generate *in silico* data and drive experimentation toward novel and unforeseen directions. In addition, in recent years, high-throughput RNA sequencing (RNA-Seq) is rapidly emerging as a powerful platform for more accurate quantitative transcriptome profiling [1,2]. The advances in computational power and technological capabilities have enabled faster processing time and lower cost for generation of RNA-Seq data. Compared to expression microarrays, RNA-Seq has considerable advantages including the detection of novel transcripts and isoforms, measurement of allele-specific expression, and large dynamic range of expression levels [3]. However, the large-scale volume and complexity of raw sequencing reads pose major challenges in the read alignment, transcript assembly, transcript quantification, normalization, as well as differential expression analysis [4]. To address these issues, software tools have been developed, refined, and optimized, mainly focusing on accuracy,

Computational Immunology: Models and Tools. DOI: http://dx.doi.org/10.1016/B978-0-12-803697-6.00007-2

efficiency, processing speed, and statistical computation. Furthermore, scientists have designed a cloud-based workflow platform that enables reliable and scalable data analysis, particularly in conjunction with commercial cloud services. The use of cloud-computing services relieves the burden of investing substantial hardware infrastructures and skilled informatics support at a modest cost. Hence, RNA-Seq data, a widely used alternative to expression microarrays, is the driving force toward better, more efficient platforms and frameworks for analysis of high-dimensional genetic data. In addition to tools and techniques, pipelines for RNA-Seq analysis have also been especially useful in many studies. For instance, *Galaxy* (https://usegalaxy.org/) provides a comprehensive collection of tools for automatic data analysis, including analysis of RNA-Seq data, with a user-friendly web interface [5]. Due to the limited resources, many historical studies were designed based on single time point RNA-Seq. However, over the past few years, with the advances of computational power and reduced cost of data generation, more and more time course experimental data are becoming available [6,7]. In fact, for modeling purposes and *in silico* experimentation, time course experimental data is especially valuable and the need for time-course data dictates the types of experimental designs. Such rich data can be used to infer network topologies as well as to calibrate complex networks that are in turn very useful in generating model-driven hypothesis that can be used effectively to guide experimental design (Chapter 4). Furthermore, as new datasets and metadata are emerging more frequently than analytical tools, it is important to develop statistical as well as analytical strategies that are versatile and can be adopted to a wide range of applications in a timely manner.

This chapter will highlight the value of rich data and specially time course data and the importance of metadata, especially for large and complex dataset. The chapter will also focus on different tools, pipelines, and techniques essential to translate high-dimensional data to computational models and finally to *in silico* experimentation and hypothesis generation (Figure 7.1).

BIG BATA DRIVES BIG MODELS

In recent years, high-throughput RNA-Seq has rapidly emerged as a powerful and versatile platform for more precise quantitative transcriptome profiling [1,2]. The technological advances in automated DNA sequencing has enabled RNA-Seq data generation with faster

The sequencing-modeling pipeline

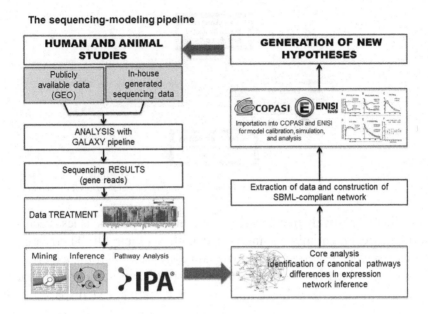

Figure 7.1 Sequencing to modeling pipeline.

processing time and lower cost. Compared to expression microarrays, RNA-Seq has considerable advantages including the detection of novel transcripts and isoforms, measurement of allele-specific expression, and large dynamic range of expression levels [3]. However, the large-scale volume and complexity of raw sequencing reads pose major challenges in the read alignment, transcript assembly, gene or transcript quantification, normalization, and differential expression analysis [4]. To tackle these issues, many software tools have been developed, focusing on improved performance in terms of accuracy, efficiency, processing speed, and statistical computation. For some steps in the pipeline of RNA-Seq data analysis that consume large processing time and memory, tools may have a capability to provide multi-processor support (e.g., *TopHat2*) [8]. Furthermore, scientists have designed cloud-based workflow platforms that enable reliable and scalable data analysis, particularly in conjunction with commercial cloud services. These advances and higher computational power have allowed design and implementation of time course experiments more feasible.

However, even though richer datasets are becoming widespread, the immunology experiments are still very costly, yet they provide more accurate and informative outcome. In contrast, computational

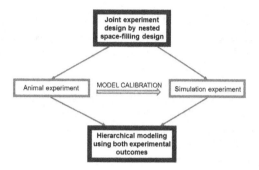

Figure 7.2 Joint experimental design and modeling for immunology experiment and simulation experiment.

modeling is relatively inexpensive; however, the outcome is less accurate and can be potentially contaminated with artifacts [9]. Therefore, to bridge knowledge extraction more seamlessly we design the experimental settings jointly for both immunology experiments and computational modeling studies. To achieve this goal, we develop a nested space-filling design [10] with the accommodation of both quantitative and qualitative factors. The nested structure design enables a small space-filling design to be embedded into a large space-filling design. Then the small design is used for the animal experiment and the large design is used for the simulation experiments. Under this strategy, the outcomes from the immunology experiments can be used to calibrate the simulation model effectively. Moreover, we adopt a hierarchical modeling strategy [11] for the calibrated simulation model to obtain accurate parameter estimation. It will lead to a more precise sensitive analysis for identifying significant factors, and hence discovering critical regions for optimal matching of the experimental data. Figure 7.2 illustrates the idea of joint experimental design between wet-lab studies and modeling through an iterative cycle.

Experimental Planning and Power Analysis

RNA-Seq is the process of using next-generation sequencing (NGS) technique to reveal a snapshot of RNA presence and quantity from a genome at a given moment in time. Although the cost of NGS has been reduced significantly as the technology advances, it remains critical to have an efficient experimental design and analysis for the detection of significant gene expression in RNA-Seq [12]. In such experimental planning, both the number of biological replicates and the depth of sequencing are critical factors to analyze. Several studies have investigated the experimental design for RNA-Seq with respect to the use of replicates, sample size, and sequencing depth [12–15]. In general, estimating the power and optimal sample size for the RNA-Seq differential expression tests is challenging because there may not be analytical solutions for RNA-Seq sample size and power calculations [16,17]. Numerical methods such as Monte Carlo simulations have been employed for the power analysis [18,19]. There are also several works investigating differences between statistical packages of RNA-Seq DE analysis [12,20–22]. In our work, we use a comprehensive power analysis through the simulation model to fully understand the magnitude of differential expression in terms of the sample size and sequencing depth. The major advantage of the simulation is that outcomes can be studied that are timely with flexible number of replicates. Hence it is possible to conduct the hypothesis testing [23] and assess the contingency table [24] under various experimental settings *in silico*. Considering the two-way layout [25] as an illustration example, we assume equal sample size n for each level combination. By systematically varying the value of n and the value of sequencing depth h, we respectively generate the simulation data from the simulation model, and calculate the performance measures including true positive rate (TPR), false positive rate (FPR), and false discovery rate [26]. Then, the quantity of performance measure can be expressed as a function of n and h, leading to a full scope of the detection effectiveness under different analysis techniques such as DESeq [27] and NBPSeq [28]. Figure 7.3 illustrates the idea of the proposed power analysis on FPR at different sample size and sequencing depth. Based on the fitted FPR surface, it is possible to predict the detection performance with unknown values of sample size and sequencing depth. Moreover, the confidence band of the FPR surface can also be obtained by analyzing the multiple simulated experimental outcomes generated from the simulation model. Therefore, such a framework can effectively evaluate the efficiency of the experimental design strategy, and consequently finds the optimal strategy of design planning to achieve high testing power on the detection of differential expression.

RNA-Seq Analysis Pipeline

Typically, read mapping is the most computationally challenging step in the RNA-Seq analysis (Figure 7.4). *TopHat* is a popular tool designed to align RNA-Seq reads to a genome using *Bowtie* and to identify splice junctions without a reference annotation, thereby

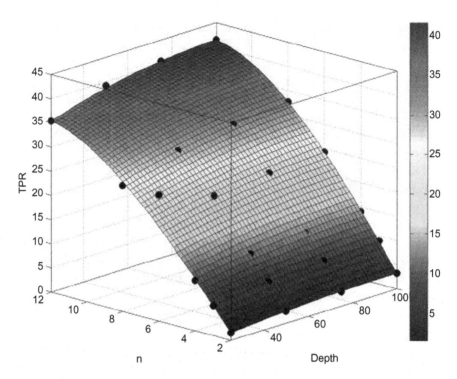

Figure 7.3 An illustration of the proposed power analysis on FPR at different sample size and sequencing depth. The FPR is calculated under the data with n = 2, 3, 4, 6, 8, 12 *and* h = 25%, 50%, 75%, 100%. *The surface is fitted using polynomial basis functions.*

having the capability of detecting new splice junctions [29]. Compared to previous RNA-Seq splice detection methods, *TopHat* has shown a significant advancement in its performance and efficiency. Recently, a new version of *TopHat* called *TopHat2* has been released with significant enhancements over *TopHat* and the increased ability to align RNA-Seq reads [8]. *TopHat2* provides support for *Bowtie2* and its own indel-finding algorithm that increases the indel-finding ability of *Bowtie2*. Some major features introduced in *TopHat2* are: (1) *TopHat2* can deal with more types of sequencing data including ABI SOLiD data, (2) it can handle reads of various lengths, allowing for merging datasets with different lengths, and (3) it can align reads across fusion breaks. The same research group that has developed the *TopHat* series designed a fast spliced aligner, *HISAT*, using a novel hierarchical indexing strategy that employs two types of indexes for spliced alignment based on the Burrows−Wheeler transform and the Ferragina−Manzini index [30].

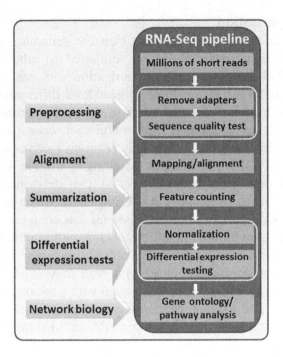

Figure 7.4 Overview of a typical RNA-Seq analysis pipeline.

One of the key advantages of this algorithm is that it uses a modest amount of random access memory with equal or better accuracy than other existing methods, enabling users to run their tasks in a single conventional computer. *STAR* was developed to overcome the drawbacks of existing aligners including high mapping error rate, low speed, and read length limitation [31]. *STAR* is capable of handling both long and short RNA-Seq data and of running parallel threads on multicore systems. In a systematic evaluation of spliced alignment programs, *STAR* demonstrated increased alignment precision and sensitivity, and significantly improved mapping speed [32]. Wu and Nacu designed a method called *GSNAP* to detect short- and long-distance splicing using probabilistic models of donor and acceptor splice sites or a database of known exon−intron sites, fulfilling both mapping speed and sensitivity needed in the detection of complex variants and splicing [33]. Wang et al. [34] developed a splice discovery method called *MapSplice* that has high sensitivity and specificity in detecting splice junctions using efficient approximate sequence alignment methods, resulting in improved central processing unit (CPU) and memory efficiency.

Read Summarization

Read summarization is an essential step for genomic analysis using RNA-Seq mapping data. However, compared to other steps in the RNA-Seq workflow, the read summarization step has received relatively little attention [35,36]. Prior to gene-level differential expression analysis, it is necessary for each gene to count the number of aligned reads that overlap its exons [35]. A useful tool, *htseq-count*, has been designed for this purpose [35,36]. This program receives a SAM/BAM file and a GTF/GFF file as input, resulting in a table with counts of aligned reads in a gene level. Liao et al. [36] developed an efficient tool, *featureCounts*, to quantify RNA-Seq reads, which is significantly faster than existing algorithms and uses far less computer memory by using chromosome hashing, feature blocking, and multithreading techniques. However, these methods do not address some issues that are commonly found in the mapping: (1) a read may align with multiple locations (multireads), (2) reads may align with positions where several genes overlap, and (3) alignments may span exon junctions. To solve these problems, *Rcount* was developed. *Rcount* also has the ability of assigning priorities to certain feature types and of editing the genome annotation [37].

Differential Expression Analysis

One of the fundamental processes in RNA-Seq analysis is to investigate whether counts for genomic features such as exons, genes, or transcripts that were quantified in the read summarization step are significantly different across experimental conditions. The count is mainly attributable to technical biases by library preparation protocols and sequencing platforms [22]. To this end, researchers have developed normalization methods for accurate comparisons between sample groups. The first normalization method named reads per kilobase per million reads (*RPKM*) was proposed by Mortazavi et al. [38] using an intuitive normalization approach that divides the gene read count by the total number of reads (in million) and gene length (in kilobase). Trapnell et al. [4] designed a variation of *RPKM* called fragments per kilobase of exon per million mapped reads (*FPKM*) to accommodate pair-end reads. However, *RPKM* and *FPKM* methods may perform poorly when highly differentially expressed genes exist and it is difficult to handle the normalized counts statistically [39]. To overcome these issues, more advanced methods for differential expression analysis have been developed. These methods have their own normalization algorithms. Robinson et al. developed a software package, *edgeR* for a flexible and powerful analysis using several statistical methods including negative binomial model to intuitively separate biological from technical variation, empirical Bayes to estimate gene-specific variability even when relatively few replicate samples are available, and generalized linear model to accommodate arbitrarily complex experiments [40−42]. Anders and Huber [27] extended the negative binomial distribution−based model used in *edgeR*, which is called *DESeq*, with more general, data-driven relationships of variance and mean, resulting in models with better fits. Recently, the same research group presented a new version of *DESeq* called *DESeq2* with several novel features that enable to improve stability and interpretability of analysis results using shrinkage estimators for dispersion and fold change compared to maximum likelihood−based solutions [43]. Hardcastle and Kelly designed an empirical Bayesian-based algorithm, *baySeq*, that enables to perform more complex experimental designs and to simultaneously establish posterior probabilities of multiple models that define patterns of differential expression. Using simulation and real data, they demonstrated that this method can achieve equivalent or improved performance compared to existing algorithms [44]. Wang et al. [45] introduced a Poisson distribution−based approach, *DEGseq*, that produces a text file that includes statistic values for each gene and an XHTML summary page. Trapnell et al. [46] designed a highly accurate differential expression tool, *Cuffdiff*, that incorporates both cross-replicate biological and technical variability. Unlike other methods mentioned above, *Cuffdiff* calculates differential expression *p*-values based on *FPKM*. *Cufflinks* reconstructs the transcripts and isoforms using the reads mapped by *TopHat*. *Cuffcompare* is used for comparison of assembled transcripts with a reference (Figure 7.5).

Time Series Data

Expression profiling over time provides a rich overview of the dynamical behavior of the system and can be very valuable source of knowledge and could also be used for calibration of computational models. However, extracting insightful information from such data is a daunting task. Different methods have been developed to address a variety of questions. In 2005, Storey et al. [47] proposed a significant method for analyzing time course microarray studies; the method can analyze time series microarray data in order to assess the differential expression from whole time series as opposed to the traditional

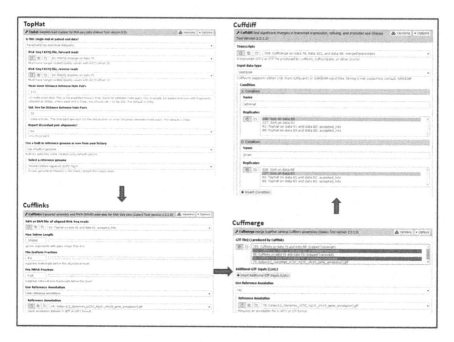

Figure 7.5 TopHat–Cufflinks–Cuffcompare–Cuffdiff *pipeline for RNA-Seq analysis in* Galaxy.

methods where each time points are analyzed independently. In 2010 [48], a novel method was developed to model temporal gene expression in order to identity key time intervals during which each gene would be differentially expressed; the approach was based on Gaussian process regression. That work was further expanded [49] to study multiple time course experiments that are condition specific. Combining differentially regulated transcriptional profiles with transcription factor binding site and pathway information was a key to identify previously known and new putative transcriptional mechanisms involved in CD4+ T-cell subset differentiation. The framework is applicable to quantify differential time course dynamics of many types of datasets and generalizes to any number of conditions. In 2013, Zaslavsky et al. [50] developed TIDAL (*TIme Dependent Activity Linker*), a software solution for the identification of transcriptional network that drives expression changes. The input to TIDAL consists of gene expression time series; however, internally, the tool makes use of TRANSFAC transcription factor binding site descriptions and genomic multiple alignments with transcription start site annotations for transcription factor binding site filtering. More recently, additional refined methods have been proposed, such as *maSigPro* [51,52]. For instance, *maSigPro* takes into account the temporal correlation and therefore would make it possible to carry out more detailed analysis of the observed dynamics, including quantification of similarities and differences between the observed kinetics. The system is designed for the analysis of transcriptomic time courses. It models gene expression by polynomial regression and identifies expression changes along one or across several time series. The method progresses in two regression steps: selecting genes with non-flat profiles and creating best regression models for each gene with variable profile. The method [51,52] was developed to treat continuous microarray intensities and was updated to be used for RNA-Seq count data by incorporating generalized linear models. Finally, in a recent review [53], current methods for identification of temporal changes in gene expression using RNA-Seq are discussed. The majority of the methods are limited to static pairwise comparison of time points; however, very few are focusing on temporal dynamics and or specific to RNA-Seq data types. These methods are continuously being developed and refined, but the field is still in its infancy and further development is needed to bridge the gap between data production and usage.

In essence, only a handful of tools and techniques have been specifically tailored to analyze the time series RNA-Seq data [51,54−57]. In some instances, tools that have been previously developed for other types of data have been redesigned for RNA-Seq data [51]. In addition, as technology evolves with new methods and new datasets emerging more frequently than analytical tools, it is important to develop strategies that are versatile and can be adapted to a wide range of applications. A strategy that is simple, yet powerful and scalable and that can be adapted to many data types could significantly reduce the time needed to adjust tools for new data as they become available and widely used. The technological advances that can be easily fine-tuned, modified, and used for different applications are fundamental to help bridge the gap between "big data" production and knowledge consumption.

We have developed an adaptive robust analytical strategy to analyze high-dimensional time series data, along with a multistage clustering technique. The first method is unsupervised, while the second is a supervised method, but both approaches can be used to analyze an RNA-Seq time course experiment and give a different perspective on the same dataset. The methods are based on an initial statistical analysis for the identification of significant genes. The presented methods focus on a dynamical analysis of the significant genes identified using a statistical approach, such as ANOVA.

Both presented approaches are unique for their flexibility, scalability, and efficiency. They are presented as a method that can be applied to RNA-Seq time series data, but the strategies can be easily customized for other time series data types.

Unsupervised High-Resolution Clustering

This strategy is based on creating a library of expression pattern motifs. The patterns are constructed based on predefined building blocks that would represent the expression pattern for different combinations at different expression levels (for instance, *basal level, and high level of expression*). Each pattern of expression will be ranked with respect to each motif in the library using a distance measure such as cosine similarity score. The analysis can reveal the most recurrent temporal motifs within different datasets. In addition, each pattern in the library can be compared to all other patterns and similar patterns can be grouped into very large-scale datasets. However, we predict that only a small number of patterns will be detected for each condition, and that representative set defines the *dynamical signature* for that condition. Gene ontology (GO) can then be performed on the genes for each of the identified patterns to highlight synchronized common functionalities and processes. Figure 7.6 highlights the key steps of the

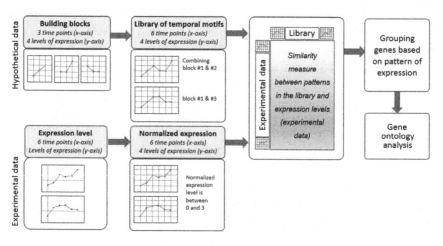

Figure 7.6 Unsupervised high-resolution clustering to identify dynamical signature set.

process. In essence, this unsupervised approach will underline the key functions and group genes based on their temporal behavior and provide a framework to analyze and compare different mechanism of action under various conditions. Furthermore, the temporal analysis can be used to further investigate genes or transcripts that are less studied by placing them in the context of well-characterized genes.

Supervised Multistage Clustering to Cluster Genes Based on Pattern of Expression

This strategy is based on fuzzy c-mean clustering techniques in combination with GO analysis. The iterative process—*multistage*—will ensure that the number of clusters is adequate for the size and characteristics of the dataset. This method will focus on biologically relevant assumptions to group time series data into different groups based on their pattern of expression. A similar approach was used in a recent study [6] to analyze time course RNA-Seq data for the study of Th17 cell differentiation. Similarly, multistage clustering in a new study [58] was used to identify clusters in multidimensional space through recursion with the goal of identifying, organizing, and understanding large biological datasets. Our method is a hybrid of these two approaches, where each subcluster will be mapped to functional group to discover novel function for uncharacterized or less studied genes. At the core of this analysis lies the assumption that gene expression can be unchanged, up-regulated, or down-regulated (thus three initial clusters). The three initial clusters can be further classified and fine-tuned based on the number of genes in the cluster, the patterns of expression of the genes, and the GO classification for the genes in the cluster. The multistage process will group genes based on the timing of their pattern of expression as well as the level of their expression. Furthermore, GO classification can be used to identify the optimal number of clusters that is biologically relevant. Finally, through this iterative data-driven process, the less informative genes are clustered together and can be filtered out in the process, making the analysis for large gene set slightly easier. An average P-value obtained from the ANOVA analysis further indicates the level of significance for each cluster.

These methods have the potential to be transformative as they can translate a differentially expressed gene list to function and further enhance our understanding of biological processes that are driving the immune response to a specific treatment. These analyses are rich as they provide a temporal view of the varying processes and can be instrumental in identifying timing and dosages of treatment regimens for clinical purposes. Furthermore, the outcome of these analytical procedures can be channeled to build computational models that can be used for generating model-driven hypothesis and strengthening the overall knowledge discovery (KD) process.

TOOLS, TECHNIQUES, AND PIPELINES

RNA-Seq Analysis in the Cloud

The emergence of NGS technologies has revolutionized molecular biology with significantly improved high-throughput sequencing data. However, the increasing volume of sequencing data poses a practical challenge for storing and processing such large-scale data in a local environment, thereby requiring powerful frameworks for computational analysis and efficient data management. Cloud-computing platforms have received a great deal of attention as a solution for these issues. Several commercial or noncommercial cloud platforms have been built including Amazon Elastic Compute Cloud (Amazon EC2), Elastic MapReduce (Amazon EMR), IBM/Google Cloud Computing University Initiative, and Magellan funded by the US Department of Energy. Hong et al. [59] developed a user-friendly RNA-Seq analysis tool called *FX* that can be run on the local Hadoop systems as well as Amazon EC2. In this system, reads are aligned onto known transcripts generated from mRNA sequences of RefSeq, UCSC, and Ensembl databases and the remaining unmapped reads are aligned onto the human genome reference. This approach can reduce the misalignment of reads that can be caused by splicing junctions. Sreedharan et al. [60] presented an open-source online platform called *Oqtans* that facilitates quantitative RNA-Seq analysis and allows for customizable and extended analysis workflows by integrating into the *Galaxy* framework. *Oqtans* provides an interface with *topGO* for enriched GO analysis for differentially expressed genes [61]. Zhao et al. [3] developed *Stormbow*, a cloud-based software package that is connected with Amazon Web Services, which enables a scalable and cost-effective large-scale RNA-Seq data analysis. Langmead et al. designed *Myrna*, a cloud-computing pipeline for RNA-Seq differential expression analysis. *Myrna* can be run on Amazon EMR, on any Hadoop cluster, or on a single computer [62]. Afgan et al. introduced a cloud resource management system called *Galaxy CloudMan* that facilitates managing cloud-computing resources with preconfigured tools needed for RNA-Seq analysis on Amazon EC2 [63,64]. Access to these tools is handled through *Galaxy* that provides a web-based integrated analysis environment and graphical user interface. *CloudMan* also provides a simple web-based interface to manage cloud resources and to access the *Galaxy* interface.

The large volume and complexity of RNA-Seq data has accelerated the development of many algorithms and tools needed for each step of RNA-Seq analysis pipeline, considering the improved performance in the following criteria: processing time, use of memory and CPU, accuracy, and reproducibility. The development of such methods that meet these criteria necessitates a high-level statistics, programming, and algorithm design techniques. Even if numerous tools for RNA-Seq analysis have been designed, there is a paucity of programs enabling a higher-level analysis of regulatory networks and simulations.

RNA Rocket at the PAThosystems Resource Integration Center

Many potential users of RNA-Seq workflows are limited not only by access to high-performance computational resources, as already noted, they can also be informatics-naïve and may not have bioinformatics staff on hand to assist with such analyses. For example, the infectious disease research communities typically have many pathogen genomes because of the relatively small genome sizes (as compared to mammals), yet their capacity to use and interpret RNA-Seq experiments is often limited. To address such challenges requires the development of software services for informatics-naïve users. Experience has shown, from bacterial genome annotation, that such automated systems can be very beneficial in increasing throughput and access to bioinformatics analysis for broader communities of typical bench biologist users, many of whom are generating much of the data (e.g., see RAST [65]). The PAThosystems Resource Integration Center (PATRIC, www.patricbrc.org), a NIAID-funded Bioinformatics Resource Center for bacterial genomes [66], has addressed these user communities by developing and deploying a system, called RNA-Rocket [67]. Bacterial RNA-Seq experiments also produce large datasets, much like with eukaryotes, yet most tools for RNA-Seq analysis have been developed with eukaryotic species in mind. Bacterial transcription, however, has some significant biological properties that differentiate it from eukaryotic systems, such as the existence of overlapping genes, polycistronic messages, and lack of splice variants. Gene models for eukaryotic genes are thus not optimal for prokaryote transcripts.

RNA-Rocket, like RAST, is based on submitting data to the system and retrieving automated analysis results. Setting up an RNA-Rocket submission in PATRIC involves simple steps with simple interfaces. First, users upload data into a private workspace. They then select a strategy from two current strategies: Rockhopper (developed for bacteria) [68] or Tuxedo (developed for eukaryotes but usable on bacteria). Next, the user selects a reference genome for mapping reads. This reference genome can be either a public PATRIC genome (all eubacterial public genomes are contained and continuously updated in PATRIC using a standardized RAST annotation for comparisons), or it can be one of the user's private genomes in that they can upload into their private workspace. Then, the user can create or select an output folder in their workspace and finally, create conditions and associate them to sets of reads. Figure 7.7 shows an example of the simple submission/upload interface.

During the execution of the RNA-Rocket service, reads are aligned to a reference genome, counts are normalized across experiments, transcripts are assembled and transcript boundaries are identified, transcript abundance is quantified, tests for differential gene expression are performed, operon structures are predicted, and results are formatted for visualization in a genome browser (Figure 7.8).

Transcripts are output from the analysis. The output contains structural information such as: transcription start and stop and translation start and stop. The output also contains functional information such as gene product and gene synonyms. Importantly, since PATRIC contains all public eubacterial genomes, the output contains cross-references to the PATRIC databases containing contig identifiers and gene identifiers. Additionally, the output contains relative abundance measures of the transcripts and q-values for the differentially expressed transcripts.

As PATRIC (more details can be found in Chapter 4) is a public resource that grows exponentially in data content, it is important to provide simple ways for users to integrate their results with the public data in PATRIC for comparative analyses. The differential expression import service transforms and integrates differential expression data for viewing in PATRIC. The data can be generated by the PATRIC

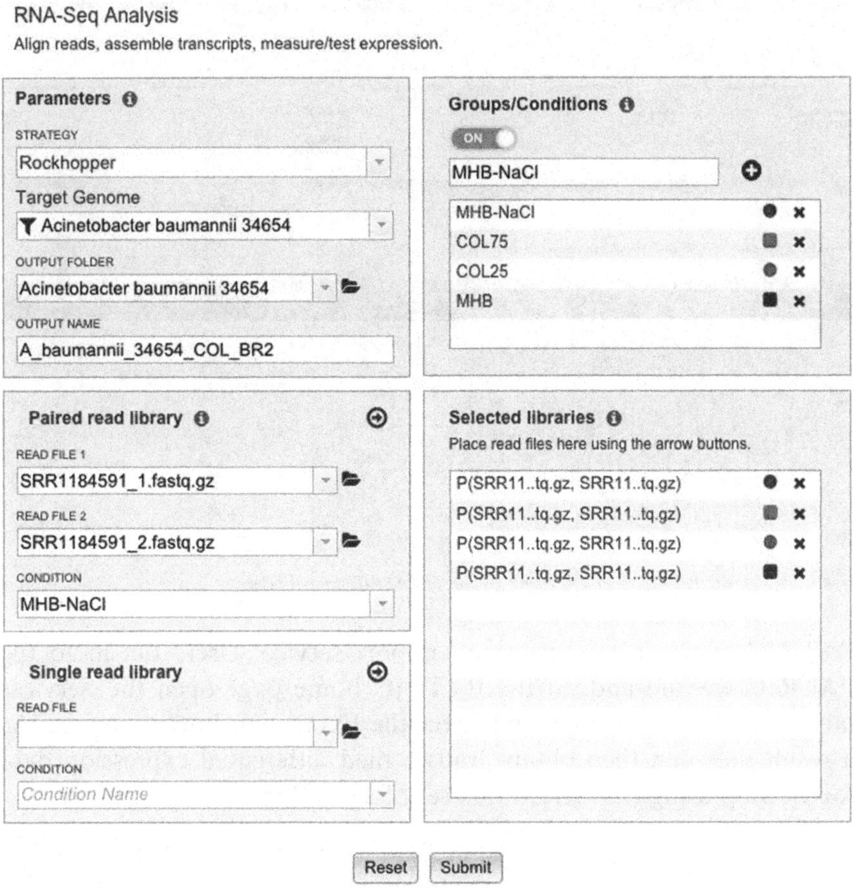

RNA-Seq Analysis

Align reads, assemble transcripts, measure/test expression.

Parameters ⓘ

STRATEGY

| Rockhopper | ▾ |

Target Genome

| ▼ Acinetobacter baumannii 34654 | ▾ |

OUTPUT FOLDER

| Acinetobacter baumannii 34654 | ▾ 📁 |

OUTPUT NAME

| A_baumannii_34654_COL_BR2 |

Groups/Conditions ⓘ

ON ⬤

| MHB-NaCl | ⊕ |

MHB-NaCl	● ✕
COL75	■ ✕
COL25	● ✕
MHB	■ ✕

Paired read library ⓘ   ➔

READ FILE 1

| SRR1184591_1.fastq.gz | ▾ 📁 |

READ FILE 2

| SRR1184591_2.fastq.gz | ▾ 📁 |

CONDITION

| MHB-NaCl | ▾ |

Single read library   ➔

READ FILE

| | ▾ 📁 |

CONDITION

| *Condition Name* | ▾ |

Selected libraries ⓘ

Place read files here using the arrow buttons.

P(SRR11..tq.gz, SRR11..tq.gz)	● ✕
P(SRR11..tq.gz, SRR11..tq.gz)	■ ✕
P(SRR11..tq.gz, SRR11..tq.gz)	● ✕
P(SRR11..tq.gz, SRR11..tq.gz)	■ ✕

[Reset] [Submit]

Figure 7.7 RNA-Rocket in PATRIC submission interface. In this execution of the service, we are using data generated at UMD on Acinetobacter baumannii *and downloaded from the SRA. While biological replicates exist, we are simplifying things for this example. The conditions are: MHB = Meuller Hinton Broth and represents "normal" growth conditions; MHB = NaCl = Meuller Hinton Broth and 200 mM NaCl. This should invoke an osmotic stress response. COL25 = 25% MIC of polymyxin-b (a natural bacteriocide found in topical creams such as Neosporin) and COL75 = 75% MIC of polymyxin-b. The reference genome is* Acinetobacter baumannii *34654, a public genome in PATRIC.*

RNA-Seq service using any of the strategies. The data can be generated using other chip-based technologies using external software. Differential expression objects are created in the user's workspace, which can be saved from one session to the next. Finally, differential expression objects contain expression data from different conditions.

In some cases, users have their own differential expression data that they have generated outside of their PATRIC workspace. In this case,

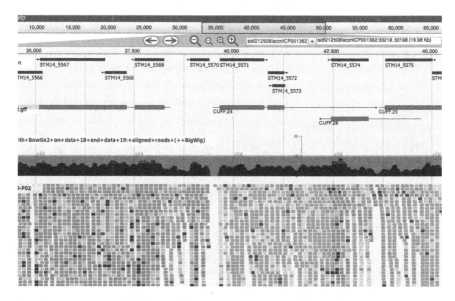

Figure 7.8 Mapping RNA reads to a reference genome in PATRIC genome browser.

PATRIC provides an expression import service. Users log in to the PATRIC website and on the PATRIC home page open the Services tab at the top of the page and select the Expression Import service. As a result they can then obtain transformed differential expression data for viewing using PATRIC's rich set of tools (Figure 7.9).

To use differential expression data in PATRIC, users can select different conditions to compare. Genes in the reference genome are displayed in a table containing: product descriptions, number of comparisons, in how may comparisons the gene was up-regulated, and in how many comparisons the gene was down-regulated. The output table can be filtered using the log ratio or Z-score that reduces the set of genes being displayed to those passing the filtering criteria. The output table can be filtered using text terms such as "transcription," for example. Finally, in addition to tabular views with data, a "heatmap" view can also be invoked (Figure 7.10).

Network Inference and Analytics

IPA: Ingenuity Pathway Analysis (IPA) software, licensed by Ingenuity Systems (Redwood City, CA), uses a database for human genes/proteins, created from manually curated literature searches (Ingenuity® ExpertAssist Findings). IPA also includes interaction

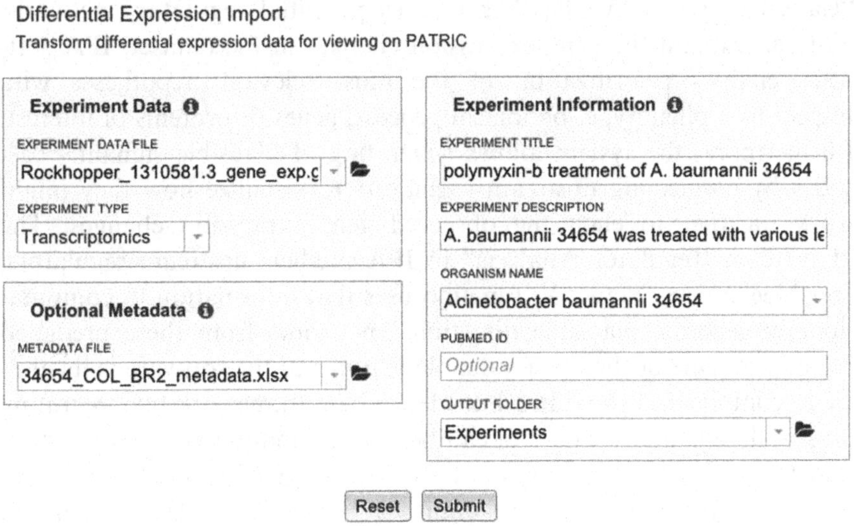

Differential Expression Import

Transform differential expression data for viewing on PATRIC

Experiment Data ⓘ

EXPERIMENT DATA FILE

Rockhopper_1310581.3_gene_exp.c ▾ 📂

EXPERIMENT TYPE

Transcriptomics ▾

Optional Metadata ⓘ

METADATA FILE

34654_COL_BR2_metadata.xlsx ▾ 📂

Experiment Information ⓘ

EXPERIMENT TITLE

polymyxin-b treatment of A. baumannii 34654

EXPERIMENT DESCRIPTION

A. baumannii 34654 was treated with various le

ORGANISM NAME

Acinetobacter baumannii 34654 ▾

PUBMED ID

Optional

OUTPUT FOLDER

Experiments ▾ 📂

Reset   Submit

Figure 7.9 Differential Expression Import Service output in PATRIC.

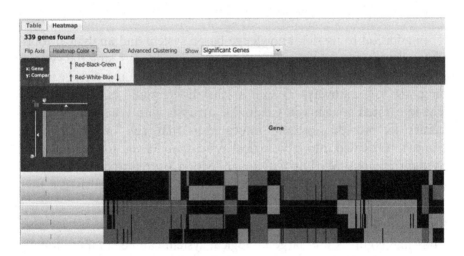

Figure 7.10 Heatmap view of expression results in PATRIC.

data from third-party databases, such as IntAct, BIND, DIP, MINT, MIPS, BIOGRID, and COGNIA. In addition, the software offers several major functional blocks, including analysis of protein–protein interaction networks, metabolomics analysis, toxicity and biomarker identification, comparative analysis for identification of changes in biological states across experimental conditions, etc. IPA can be used to guide modeling efforts and identify key pathways. For instance, the

"Causal Network Analysis" generates potential regulatory networks that can explain the gene expression changes in the dataset. IPA software enables prioritization of the most relevant hypotheses with respect to a phenotype, biological process, genes or proteins of interest. Furthermore, the system allows generating of plausible signaling cascades by connecting upstream regulators to visualize how they might work together to elicit the observed gene expression changes. The "Upstream Regulator Analysis" in IPA predicts upstream regulators, and Mechanistic Networks function uses that information to computationally generate plausible directional networks from these predicted regulators. One of the most valuable features of the software is its ability to compile and provide a knowledge base framework by integrating diverse data sources. The tool can be used to analyze and identify relationships, mechanisms, functions, and pathways of a biological system of interest from the different datasets. Furthermore, the system can also be used to build a better picture from the data. Currently species supported by IPA include human, mouse, rat, and canine; additional species are supported via ortholog mapping.

In addition to its rich knowledge based system and analytical tools, IPA software provides also visualization capabilities. Using the system, it is possible to effectively visualize and highlight the trends in the data, the key pathways as well as the differentially expressed genes. The integrated system will streamline analysis with visualization capabilities to provide accurate information that can be meticulously curated, translated into a biological system model via, for example, the Systems Biology Markup Language (SBML) for further explorations *in silico*, including methods such as supervised machine learning.

Supervised Machine Learning Methods

Modeling complex and large biological system can be computationally expensive; however, in cases where sufficient data are available, supervised machine learning techniques from artificial intelligence can be designed and optimized to build reliable yet scalable models. We have demonstrated [69–71] that Artificial Neural Networks (ANN) as well as Random Forest (RF) algorithms are efficient modeling tools as they can reduce the complexity of intracellular network models by focusing on input and output entities. We have optimized and evaluated ANN and RF algorithms using the CD4+ T-cell differentiation model [72]. The ANN and RF showed comparable performance; however, ANN was faster than RF to predict output cytokine concentrations based on input cytokines. Using supervised learning methods can provide a realistic approach for modeling complex systems when sufficient experimental data is available. To further corroborate the reliability of this approach, we have successfully tested the quality of the models by (i) performing 10-fold cross validation, (ii) challenging the model to reproduce published experimental data [73−75], and (iii) analyzing the simulation results by using data with added noise. We have shown that the trained models can be reliable and efficiently used to gain a deeper understanding of the complex interplay between different related entities.

NetGenerator

The general nonlinear dynamics can be described by a set of first-order time-invariant ordinary differential equations, initial conditions, and time range. Since the core mechanism is based on linear modeling, the differential equation system can be modified resulting in the linear state-space equation system. The NetGenerator algorithm is a heuristic approach, which is based on the observation that in gene-regulatory networks the number of connections is much lower than all possible connections. The network can be considered as a hierarchical structure originating from the input. The NetGenerator algorithm implements both observations by an iterative development of the state-space system by including coupled submodels for each time series based on a structure optimization iteratively increasing the number of connections (Figure 7.11) [76]. In addition, the NetGenerator algorithm provides two modes for integration of prior knowledge about connections of stimuli on time series, fix and flexible.

Adaptive Robust Integrative Analysis for Finding Novel Association

The effective mining of literature can provide a range of services such as hypothesis generation or finding semantic sensitive networks of association from Big Data such as PubMed—with more than 24 million citations of biomedical literature (http://www.pubmed.org/) and increasing by roughly 30,000 per day. This may also help to understand the potential confluence among different entities or concepts of interest. We have designed a fully integrated scalable text analytic tool—called Adaptive Robust Integrative Analysis for Finding Novel Association (ARIANA)—that can bridge the gap between the

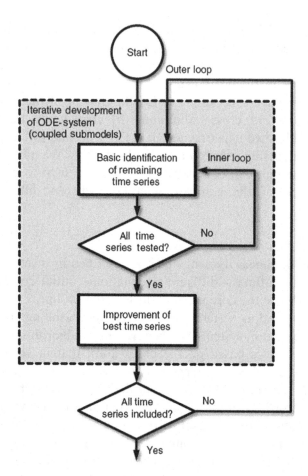

Figure 7.11 Main workflow of the NetGenerator algorithm. The outer loop iterates over all state variables, while in the inner loop the remaining time series are tested. A basic structure and parameters are identified.

"generation" and "consumption" of Big Data and increase its utility [77–80]. Traditional literature mining frameworks rely on "keyword-based approaches" and are not suitable for capturing meaningful associations to reduce the information overload or generate new hypotheses, let alone for finding networks of semantic relations. Existing techniques still lack the ability to effectively present biological data in easy-to-use form [81] to further KD by integrating heterogeneous data. To effectively reduce information overload and complement traditional means of knowledge dissemination, it is imperative to develop and use robust and scalable KD tools that are broad and resourceful enough to extract direct as well as indirect associations. The utility of such a system would be greatly enhanced with the added capability of finding semantically similar concepts related to various risk factors, side-effects, symptoms, and diseases. Using the ARIANA system we have shown that context-specific literature mining strategy can be used to find novel associations, hidden associations, and generate new hypothesis for exploratory research and collaborative studies. Using the pilot version of ARIANA [79], we were able to extract interesting knowledge, such as the association between sexually transmitted diseases and migraine, an association that published after [55] we have downloaded the abstracts from PubMed. Using the fully developed system, we were able to able to extract even more valuable information leading toward *actionable knowledge* [77,78]. The association between the drug hexamethonium and pulmonary inflammation and fibrosis was relatively unknown and related publications were also not in the database. The drug hexamethonium can be used to treat chronic hypertension of the peripheral nervous system; yet, the nonspecificity of its action led to discontinuation of its use [47,48]. However, in 2001, a healthy volunteer who was participating in an asthma study died only after few days of inhaling this drug. She was diagnosed with pulmonary inflammation and fibrosis based on chest imaging and autopsy report. [49]. This tragic accident could have been prevented if the researcher knew of a case report published in 1955 [50]; ARIANA on the other hand was able to extract this information even though the 1950 case report was not included in its database. Finally, the path from *Big Data* to *Actionable Knowledge* is multidimensional and nonlinear. However, investigation of cause–effect relationships in translational research could be a step toward bridging that gap. The modularity provided by ARIANA will further integrative analysis.

CASE STUDY: RECONSTRUCTING THE TH17 DIFFERENTIATION NETWORK

Theoretical models have been used to decipher the mechanisms controlling differentiation and function of Th17 cells by studying the relationship of RORγt with FOXP3 [82,83]. The relationship of FOXP3 and RORγt is especially important since these two transcription factors are master regulators of agonist cell differentiation programs [84,85]. On the one side, RORγt promotes pro-inflammatory secretion of IL-21 and IL-17A. On the other side, FOXP3 promotes anti-inflammatory responses through secretion of IL-10. Using computational modeling, we were able to predict and later validate the role of peroxisome proliferator activated receptor gamma (PPARγ) in modulating the plasticity between Th17 and Treg cells [72]. Due to the increasing availability of high-throughput data, combining theoretical and data-driven approaches becomes more feasible [86]. Furthermore, more recently, in a study published by Yosef et al. [6], transcriptional profiling at high temporal resolution was used to build a Th17 induction system. To build the dynamic model [87], we analyzed the data and inferred a computational modeling network using the IPA platform (see above), we translated the inferred network into a SBML-compliant system, imported the network into COmplex PAthway SImulator (COPASI) [88], and calibrated the system by using the original datasets used to build the dynamic network model (Figure 7.12). Our *in silico* predictions about the function of NLRP3 and IL-24 during Th17 differentiation revealed a modulatory role over Th17 function. Furthermore, our local sensitivity analysis highlighted the correlations between FOXP3, CEBPB, FOSL1, IRF4, and PPARγ with IL-24, as well as the correlations of IP-10, GM-CSF, IFNγ, and IL-17A with NLRP3.

To streamline the process of model construction from high-dimensional transcriptomic data, we built a semiautomated analysis

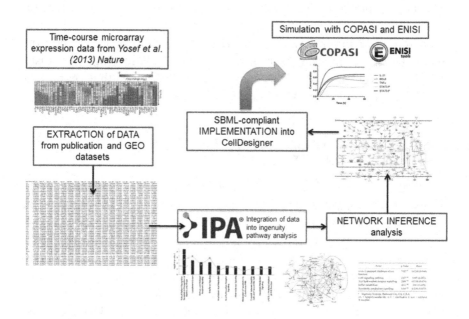

Figure 7.12 Integrated data-driven modeling pipeline.

pipeline that provides a methodological approach for dynamic model construction. First, IPA was used to identify the molecular pathways and functional groupings for significantly differentially expressed mRNAs from the Th17 differentiation data that was uploaded. Including both experimental and predicted connections, IPA provided a list of upstream activators, where the most up- and down-regulated genes could be observed and the information of such genes could be accessed. Based on the all the genes uploaded into IPA, we created a first inferred network (Figure 7.13(a)). The expression values of this first network were calculated based on single observations extracted from the dataset. Given the amount of interactions generated, 67 genes were selected

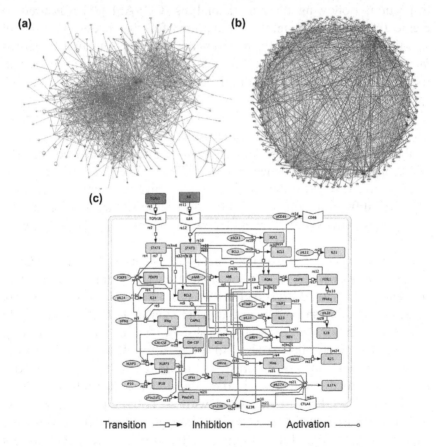

Figure 7.13 Network inference and analysis prior to importation into an SBML-compliant environment. (a) The transcriptome data was used to generate a comprehensive gene regulatory interaction network in IPA. (b) Out of all the nodes in IPA, 67 genes (up-regulated or down-regulated) were selected based on differences in expression over the Th0 compartment. (c) SBML-compliant cell designer network with a subset of genes in (b) to import into COPASI.

based on their levels of expression over the Th0 compartment (Figure 7.13(b)). Following modeling reduction to accommodate more efficient simulation capabilities, 35 genes and their interactions between them were imported them into CellDesigner (Figure 7.13(c)). This selection was performed based on inclusion of the more critical nodes to mount a Th17 differentiation cascade following IL-6 and TGF β1 induction.

The transition from a static diagram into a dynamic model of Th17 differentiation helps to not only understand the connections of the network but also observe how these connections changed over time. Furthermore, the dynamic model facilitates *in silico* experimentation than can capture novel behaviors that could not be observed by visual inspection. Following this initial analysis, COPASI [88] was used to create the ordinary differential equations for the model. The model was then calibrated using the experimental data [6]. Our first target for *in silico* experimentation was Interleukin-24 (IL-24). Upon binding to its receptors, IL-24 induces rapid activation of STAT1 and STAT3 transcription factors, both of which activate effector profiles in CD4+ T-cell differentiation [89]. The role of IL-24 during Th17 differentiation, however, is very poorly understood. The transcriptomic analysis of the Th17 differentiation datasets used in this study proved that IL-24 is highly expressed when a naïve CD4+ T cell is induced with TGFβ1 and IL-6. In order to better understand the role of IL-24 during Th17 differentiation, we performed local sensitivity analysis on the IL-24 node. Our results highlight how the increase in the initial concentration of IL-24 decreases the expression of FOXP3 and increases the expression of Th17-related molecules such as STAT3, RORc, CEBPB, and FOSL1. We further created an IL-24 null system, where the ability of IL-24 to exert its functions to other nodes was completely impaired. Results showed how the expression of FOXP3 in the IL-24 null when compared to the wild-type system remains unchanged during the approximately first 10 h. However, after 10 h, FOXP3 starts degrading over time. In contrast, in the IL-24 null system, FOXP3 reached a steady state and it did not undergo degradation. Since FOXP3 and ROR-γt are regulated with such tight balance, we next sought to determine the effect of this un-degraded FOXP3 toward the expression of RORc. Interestingly, the IL-24 null system showed less expression of RORc when compared to the wild-type Th17 model. We hypothesize that the relationship of RORc and IL-24 is FOXP3-dependent. Our results show that blocking IL-24 increases the concentration of FOXP3. The increase of FOXP3 breaks the balance of FOXP3 and RORc, which have been found to antagonize [84,85]. We also observe RORc down-regulated with the absence of IL-24. These counterintuitive results generated *in silico* by our Th17 differentiation model in regards to the role of IL-24 during Th17 induction should be validated with specific *in vitro* and *in vivo* experimental studies. Indeed, our results demonstrated that IL-24 does not correlate with IL-17A, but that it plays an important role in modulating the balance between FOXP3 and RORγt by suppressing the Treg program and induce an increase of RORc. The potential modulating role of IL-24 in the RORc−FOXP3 balance could lead to the development of IL-24 blockers as therapeutic treatment. Therefore, if these predictions were validated, IL-24 would arise as an immune-based, powerful, and potential therapeutic target to modulated inflammatory diseases characterized by a Th17 upregulation. In this case study, we established a modeling pipeline for constructing and calibrating data-driven models of Th17 differentiation. Our results highlighted the role of IL-24, SGK1, and NLRP3 as key modulators of Th17 cell differentiation. This modeling pipeline is an example of a modeling environment for building computational models with deterministic and stochastic features to generate new mechanistic immunological knowledge and to identify novel therapeutic targets for human diseases.

CONCLUDING REMARKS

A major goal of computational immunology is to construct comprehensive, multiscale network models of massively interacting systems that accurately describe the dynamics of the immune system with its effector and regulatory elements. As NGS technologies for datasets are becoming increasingly available at lower cost, the computational immunology should leverage big and complex data, along with theory to construct predictive large-scale models. These mathematical models will provide high-resolution maps for regulatory connections between intracellular and intercellular components, as well as potential new functional roles for specific genes, proteins, or metabolites. We envision that this integrative approach will be central for a general strategy toward precision medicine, suggesting alternative drugs or immune system−targeted therapy tailored specifically to an individual, and modeling-enabled safer and more effective drug discovery and development.

ACKNOWLEDGMENTS

This work was supported in part by National Institute of Allergy and Infectious Diseases Contract No. HHSN272201000056C to JBR and funds from the Nutritional Immunology and Molecular Medicine Laboratory (www.nimml.org).

REFERENCES

[1] Wang Z, Gerstein M, Snyder M. RNA-Seq: a revolutionary tool for transcriptomics. Nat Rev Genet 2009;10(1):57−63.

[2] Raghavachari N, et al. A systematic comparison and evaluation of high density exon arrays and RNA-Seq technology used to unravel the peripheral blood transcriptome of sickle cell disease. BMC Med Genomics 2012;5:28.

[3] Zhao S, Prenger K, Smith L. Stormbow: a cloud-based tool for reads mapping and expression quantification in large-scale RNA-Seq studies. ISRN bioinformatics 2013; 2013.

[4] Trapnell C, et al. Transcript assembly and quantification by RNA-Seq reveals unannotated transcripts and isoform switching during cell differentiation. Nat Biotechnol 2010;28 (5):511−15.

[5] Goecks J, et al. Galaxy: a comprehensive approach for supporting accessible, reproducible, and transparent computational research in the life sciences. Genome Biol 2010;11(8):R86.

[6] Yosef N, et al. Dynamic regulatory network controlling TH17 cell differentiation. Nature 2013;496(7446):461−8.

[7] Philipson CW, et al. Modeling the Regulatory Mechanisms by which NLRX1 Modulates Innate Immune Responses to *Helicobacter pylori* infection. PLos One 2015.

[8] Kim D, et al. TopHat2: accurate alignment of transcriptomes in the presence of insertions, deletions and gene fusions. Genome Biol 2013;14(4):R36.

[9] Santner TJ, Williams BJ, Notz WI. The design and analysis of computer experiments. New York, NY: Springer; 2003.

[10] Qian PZG, Tang B, Wu C Jeff. Nested space-filling designs for computer experiments with two levels of accuracy. Statistica Sinica 2009;19(1):287.

[11] Kennedy MC, O'Hagan A. Bayesian calibration of computer models. J R Stat Soc Series B 2001;63(3):425−64.

[12] Robles JA, et al. Efficient experimental design and analysis strategies for the detection of differential expression using RNA-sequencing. BMC Genomics 2012;13:484.

[13] Ching T, Huang S, Garmire LX. Power analysis and sample size estimation for RNA-Seq differential expression. RNA 2014;20(11):1684−96.

[14] Fang Z, Cui X. Design and validation issues in RNA-Seq experiments. Brief Bioinform 2011;12(3):280−7.

[15] Liu Y, Zhou J, White KP. RNA-Seq differential expression studies: more sequence or more replication? Bioinformatics 2014;30(3):301−4.

[16] Aban IB, Cutter GR, Mavinga N. Inferences and power analysis concerning two negative binomial distributions with an application to MRI lesion counts data. Comput Stat Data Anal 2008;53(3):820−33.

[17] Pham TV, Jimenez CR. An accurate paired sample test for count data. Bioinformatics 2012;28(18):i596−602.

[18] Srivastava S, Chen L. A two-parameter generalized Poisson model to improve the analysis of RNA-Seq data. Nucleic Acids Res 2010;38(17):e170.

[19] Vijay N, et al. Challenges and strategies in transcriptome assembly and differential gene expression quantification. A comprehensive *in silico* assessment of RNA-Seq experiments. Mol Ecol 2013;22(3):620−34.

[20] Kvam VM, Liu P, Si Y. A comparison of statistical methods for detecting differentially expressed genes from RNA-Seq data. Am J Bot 2012;99(2):248−56.

[21] Nookaew I, et al. A comprehensive comparison of RNA-Seq-based transcriptome analysis from reads to differential gene expression and cross-comparison with microarrays: a case study in *Saccharomyces cerevisiae*. Nucleic Acids Res 2012;40(20):10084−97.

[22] Rapaport F, et al. Comprehensive evaluation of differential gene expression analysis methods for RNA-Seq data. Genome Biol 2013;14(9):R95.

[23] Lehmann EL. Testing statistical hypotheses. The Wadsworth & Brooks/Cole statistics/probability series. 2nd ed. Pacific Grove, CA: Wadsworth & Brooks/Cole Advanced Books & Software; 1991. vol. xx, p. 600.

[24] Bishop YMM, Fienberg SE, Holland PW. Discrete multivariate analysis: theory and practice. Cambridge, MA: MIT Press; 1975. vol. x, p. 557.

[25] Scheffe H. The analysis of variance. Wiley publication in mathematical statistics. New York, NY: John Wiley & Sons; 1959. vol. xvi, p. 477.

[26] Benjamini Y, Hochberg Y. Controlling the false discovery rate—a practical and powerful approach to multiple testing. J R Stat Soc Series B 1995;57(1):289−300.

[27] Anders S, Huber W. Differential expression analysis for sequence count data. Genome Biol 2010;11(10):R106.

[28] Di YM, et al. The NBP negative binomial model for assessing differential gene expression from RNA-Seq. Stat Appl Genet Mol Biol 2011;10(1).

[29] Trapnell C, Pachter L, Salzberg SL. TopHat: discovering splice junctions with RNA-Seq. Bioinformatics 2009;25(9):1105−11.

[30] Kim D, Langmead B, Salzberg SL. HISAT: a fast spliced aligner with low memory requirements. Nat Methods 2015;12(4):357−60.

[31] Dobin A, et al. STAR: ultrafast universal RNA-Seq aligner. Bioinformatics 2013;29 (1):15−21.

[32] Engström PG, et al. Systematic evaluation of spliced alignment programs for RNA-Seq data. Nat Methods 2013;10(12):1185−91.

[33] Wu TD, Nacu S. Fast and SNP-tolerant detection of complex variants and splicing in short reads. Bioinformatics 2010;26(7):873−81.

[34] Wang K, et al. MapSplice: accurate mapping of RNA-Seq reads for splice junction discovery. Nucleic Acids Res 2010;38(18):e178.

[35] Anders S, Pyl PT, Huber W. HTSeq—a Python framework to work with high-throughput sequencing data. Bioinformatics 2015;31(2):166−9.

[36] Liao Y, Smyth GK, Shi W. featureCounts: an efficient general purpose program for assigning sequence reads to genomic features. Bioinformatics 2014;30(7):923−30.

[37] Schmid MW, Grossniklaus U. Rcount: simple and flexible RNA-Seq read counting. Bioinformatics 2015;31(3):436−7.

[38] Mortazavi A, et al. Mapping and quantifying mammalian transcriptomes by RNA-Seq. Nat Methods 2008;5(7):621−8.

[39] Tong P, et al. SIBER: systematic identification of bimodally expressed genes using RNAseq data. Bioinformatics 2013;29(5):605–13.

[40] Robinson MD, McCarthy DJ, Smyth GK. edgeR: a Bioconductor package for differential expression analysis of digital gene expression data. Bioinformatics 2010;26(1):139–40.

[41] McCarthy DJ, Chen Y, Smyth GK. Differential expression analysis of multifactor RNA-Seq experiments with respect to biological variation. Nucleic Acids Res 2012;40 (10):4288–97.

[42] Zhou X, Lindsay H, Robinson MD. Robustly detecting differential expression in RNA sequencing data using observation weights. Nucleic Acids Res 2014;42(11):e91.

[43] Love MI, Huber W, Anders S. Moderated estimation of fold change and dispersion for RNA-Seq data with DESeq2. Genome Biol 2014;15(12):550.

[44] Hardcastle TJ, Kelly KA. baySeq: empirical Bayesian methods for identifying differential expression in sequence count data. BMC Bioinformatics 2010;11:422.

[45] Wang L, et al. DEGseq: an R package for identifying differentially expressed genes from RNA-Seq data. Bioinformatics 2010;26(1):136–8.

[46] Trapnell C, et al. Differential analysis of gene regulation at transcript resolution with RNA-Seq. Nat Biotechnol 2013;31(1):46–53.

[47] Storey JD, et al. Significance analysis of time course microarray experiments. Proc Natl Acad Sci USA 2005;102(36):12837–42.

[48] Stegle O, et al. A robust Bayesian two-sample test for detecting intervals of differential gene expression in microarray time series. J Comput Biol 2010;17(3):355–67.

[49] Aijo T, et al. An integrative computational systems biology approach identifies differentially regulated dynamic transcriptome signatures which drive the initiation of human T helper cell differentiation. BMC Genomics 2012;13:572.

[50] Zaslavsky E, et al. Reconstruction of regulatory networks through temporal enrichment profiling and its application to H1N1 influenza viral infection. BMC Bioinformatics 2013;14 (Suppl. 6):S1.

[51] Nueda MJ, Tarazona S, Conesa A. Next maSigPro: updating maSigPro bioconductor package for RNA-Seq time series. Bioinformatics 2014;30(18):2598–602.

[52] Conesa A, Nueda M. Next-masigpro: dealing with RNA-Seq time series. EMBnet J 2013;19:42–3.

[53] Oh S, et al. The analytical landscape of static and temporal dynamics in transcriptome data. Front Genet 2014;5:35.

[54] Äijö T, et al. Methods for time series analysis of RNA-Seq data with application to human Th17 cell differentiation. Bioinformatics 2014;30(12):i113–20.

[55] Mechkarska M, et al. Host-defense peptides from skin secretions of the octoploid frogs *Xenopus vestitus* and *Xenopus wittei* (Pipidae): insights into evolutionary relationships. Comp Biochem Physiol Part D Genomics Proteomics 2014;11:20–8.

[56] Oh S, et al. Time series expression analyses using RNA-Seq: a statistical approach. Biomed Res Int 2013;2013:203681.

[57] Zou M, Conzen SD. A new dynamic Bayesian network (DBN) approach for identifying gene regulatory networks from time course microarray data. Bioinformatics 2005;21 (1):71–9.

[58] Friedman A, et al. A multistage mathematical approach to automated clustering of high-dimensional noisy data. Proc Natl Acad Sci USA 2015;112(14):4477–82.

[59] Hong D, et al. FX: an RNA-Seq analysis tool on the cloud. Bioinformatics 2012;28 (5):721–3.

[60] Sreedharan VT, et al. Oqtans: the RNA-Seq workbench in the cloud for complete and repro-ducible quantitative transcriptome analysis. Bioinformatics 2014;30(9):1300–1.

[61] Alexa A, Rahnenführer J, Lengauer T. Improved scoring of functional groups from gene expression data by decorrelating GO graph structure. Bioinformatics 2006;22(13):1600–7.

[62] Langmead B, Hansen KD, Leek JT. Cloud-scale RNA-sequencing differential expression analysis with Myrna. Genome Biol 2010;11(8):R83.

[63] Afgan E, et al. Galaxy CloudMan: delivering cloud compute clusters. BMC Bioinformatics 2010;11(Suppl. 12):S4.

[64] Afgan E, Chapman B, Taylor J. CloudMan as a platform for tool, data, and analysis distri-bution. BMC Bioinformatics 2012;13:315.

[65] Aziz RK, et al. The RAST server: rapid annotations using subsystems technology. BMC Genomics 2008;9.

[66] Wattam AR, et al. PATRIC, the bacterial bioinformatics database and analysis resource. Nucleic Acids Res 2014;42(D1):D581–91.

[67] Warren AS, et al. RNA-Rocket: an RNA-Seq analysis resource for infectious disease research. Bioinformatics 2015;31(9):1496–8.

[68] McClure R, et al. Computational analysis of bacterial RNA-Seq data. Nucleic Acids Res 2013;41(14).

[69] Lu P, et al. Supervised learning methods in modeling of CD4+ T cell heterogeneity. BioData Min 2015;8:27.

[70] Lu P, et al. Supervised learning with artificial neural networks in modeling of cell differentia-tion processes. Emerging trends in computational biology, bioinformatics and systems biol-ogy. Burlignton, MA: Morgan Kaufmann; 2015.

[71] Mei Y, et al. Neural network models for classifying immune cell subsets. Shangai, China: BIBM; 2013.

[72] Carbo A, et al. Systems modeling of molecular mechanisms controlling cytokine-driven CD4+ T cell differentiation and phenotype plasticity. PLoS Comput Biol 2013;9(4): e1003027.

[73] Matsuoka K, et al. T-bet upregulation and subsequent interleukin 12 stimulation are essen-tial for induction of Th1 mediated immunopathology in Crohn's disease. Gut 2004;53 (9):1303–8.

[74] Bettelli E, et al. Reciprocal developmental pathways for the generation of pathogenic effec-tor TH17 and regulatory T cells. Nature 2006;441(7090):235–8.

[75] McGeachy MJ, et al. TGF-beta and IL-6 drive the production of IL-17 and IL-10 by T cells and restrain T(H)-17 cell-mediated pathology. Nat Immunol 2007;8(12):1390–7.

[76] Weber M, et al. Inference of dynamical gene-regulatory networks based on time-resolved multi-stimuli multi-experiment data applying NetGenerator V2.0. BMC Syst Biol 2013;7:1.

[77] Abedi V, Yeasin M, Zand R. Literature mining and ontology mapping applied to big data. In: Akhgar B, Saathoff G, Arabnia H, Hill R, Staniforth A, Bayerl, editors. Mining big data to improve national security. Waltham, MA: Elsevier; 2015. p. 184–208.

[78] Abedi V, Yeasin M, Zand R. Empirical study using network of semantically related associa-tions in bridging the knowledge gap. J Transl Med 2014;12:324.

[79] Abedi V, Yeasin M, Zand R. ARIANA: adaptive robust and integrative analysis for finding novel associations. The 2014 international conference on advances in big data analytics. Las Vegas, NV: CSREA Press; 2014. p. 22–8.

[80] Abedi V, et al. An automated framework for hypotheses generation using literature. BioData Min 2012;5:13.

[81] Altman RB, et al. Text mining for biology—the way forward: opinions from leading scientists. Genome Biol 2008;9(Suppl. 2):S7.

[82] Hong T, et al. A mathematical model for the reciprocal differentiation of T helper 17 cells and induced regulatory T cells. PLoS Comput Biol 2011;7(7):e1002122.

[83] Mendoza L. A virtual culture of CD4+ T lymphocytes. Bull Math Biol 2013;75 (6):1012–29.

[84] Tartar DM, et al. FoxP3+ RORgammat+ T helper intermediates display suppressive function against autoimmune diabetes. J Immunol 2010;184(7):3377–85.

[85] Zhou L, et al. TGF-beta-induced Foxp3 inhibits T(H)17 cell differentiation by antagonizing RORgammat function. Nature 2008;453(7192):236–40.

[86] Carbo A, et al. Computational modeling of heterogeneity and function of CD4+ T cells. Front Cell Dev Biol 2014;2:31.

[87] Carbo A, et al. Modeling the dynamics of T helper 17 induction and differentiation. MOJ Immunol 2015;2(2).

[88] Hoops S, et al. COPASI—a COmplex PAthway SImulator. Bioinformatics 2006;22 (24):3067–74.

[89] Wang M, Liang P. Interleukin-24 and its receptors. Immunology 2005;114(2):166–70.

CHAPTER 8

Multiscale Modeling: Concepts, Technologies, and Use Cases in Immunology

Vida Abedi[1], Raquel Hontecillas[1], Adria Carbo[2], Casandra Philipson[2], Stefan Hoops[1], and Josep Bassaganya-Riera[1]

[1]Nutritional Immunology and Molecular Medicine Laboratory, Virginia Bioinformatics Institute, Virginia Tech, Blacksburg, VA, USA [2]Biotherapeutics Inc., Blacksburg, VA, USA

INTRODUCTION

Computational modeling is playing increasingly important roles in advancing a system-level mechanistic understanding of complex inter-related biological processes such as the mucosal immune system. *In silico* simulations guide and underpin experimental and clinical efforts and can advance the knowledge discovery and accelerate therapeutic development at an unprecedented rate. However, modeling complex systems such as the mucosal immune responses require multiscale modeling (MSM) frameworks spanning from cells to systems and substantial computational resources. The latter is becoming especially accessible in todays' *Big Data* era. Biological systems are inherently multiscale in nature, from molecules to tissues and from nanoseconds to a lifespan of several years. Hence, integration of multiple modeling technologies to understand immunological processes from signaling pathways within cells to lesion formation at the tissue level and towards clinical outcomes is the key to our understanding the complex system behavior and providing guidance for the modulation of the systems at multiple levels. Yet, MSM requires also integrating of not only multiple data sets but also multiple modeling technologies. These integration efforts seamlessly bring together computational and mathematical technologies with preclinical and clinical data types and health outcomes (Figure 8.1). In addition, modeling at multiscale levels requires addressing the model complexity, large parameter space for model calibration, differences in spatiotemporal scales, cellular states, and differences in computational technologies used for the

Computational Immunology: Models and Tools. DOI: http://dx.doi.org/10.1016/B978-0-12-803697-6.00008-4

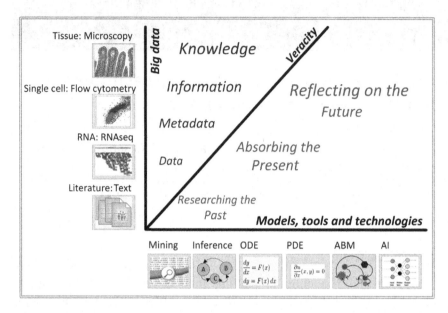

Figure 8.1 Data, tool models, and knowledge paradigm.

development of each individual scale. In this chapter, we will dissect and summarize the technical details of MSM targeted towards computational immunologists, bioinformaticians, and biologists and review the latest cutting-edge implementation of the current system in the field.

MSM CONCEPTS AND TECHNIQUES

Successful analysis of complex immune-mediated and infectious diseases requires understanding of key components at different scales *in space and time*: from molecular to tissue level and population-level scales, and from nanoseconds to years, hence the need for computational modeling across *spatiotemporal* scales. The rapid advances in computing hardware, algorithms as well as computational power have contributed to the rise of MSM; however, MSM is challenging for various reasons. MSM means (1) combining different tools, techniques, and modeling strategies; (2) integrating diverse data types at different resolution; (3) performing sensitivity analysis (SA) across scales; (4) integrating data-rich and data-poor models; (5) performing sufficiently large set of *in silico* experiments; and (6) validating the model-driven hypotheses with experimental data at the preclinical and clinical levels.

Over the last decade, an array of multiscale models was developed to empower scientists to generate novel computational hypotheses and be able to design innovative experiments to validate these hypotheses. However, although the technologies can be generalized, the MSM frameworks are usually designed for specific fields. In computational immunology, ENteric Immune Simulator (ENISI) MSM [1,2] is the first and currently the only MSM system of the mucosal immune responses. ENISI MSM prototype is specifically designed to capture four layers of spatiotemporal scales and extensible to capture other layers such as population-level health outcomes.

Although earlier modeling techniques were mainly based on a reductionist approach and models were based on the formalism of mathematical equations, recent tendencies cultivate more comprehensive and integrative approaches. Specifically, the introduction of computational systems biology and the emerging techniques from multiple disciplines such as mathematics, engineering, computer science, and artificial intelligence are the driving force towards this sudden transformative progress of computational modeling in immunology, infectious, and immune-mediated diseases. Furthermore, computational techniques can in principle capture existing knowledge into models and discover emerging behaviors and new knowledge through an iterative model analyses and simulations; however, the complex dynamics of various components and interaction between the environment and species over time makes building and calibrating comprehensive multiscale models challenging.

Modeling techniques used in MSM are mainly grouped into five main categories: deterministic models, stochastic models, logical models, rule-based models, and statistical models including parametric and nonparametric models. Each modeling framework can be best applied to a specific biological scale. For instance, modeling gene regulatory networks can be achieved by quantitative, logical, or hybrid models [3] as well as statistical models such as dynamic Bayesian network [4]; modeling intracellular phenomena, such as signaling pathways, is best achieved by utilization of ordinary differential equations (ODEs) (deterministic models) as well as stochastic models [5]; modeling intercellular processes such as cytokine and chemokine diffusion is best represented by partial differential equations (PDEs) (also deterministic models); and modeling cellular behavior is most effective if the models

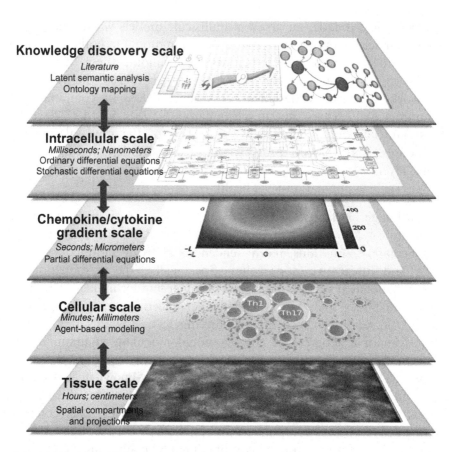

Figure 8.2 Multiscale model of the mucosal immune responses.

are developed using agent-based modeling framework (rule-based models). Finally, stochastic models can be incorporated to account for low copy number of genes, gene products, or even cell types [6].

Cohesive and robust MSM can be achieved by integrating different modeling techniques and tools into a unified modeling environment to span various spatiotemporal scales, ranging from nanometers to meters and from nanoseconds to years (see Figure 8.2). Table 8.1 summarizes the scales of spatiotemporal magnitude of ENISI MSM. At the highest level, literature mining technology, such as ARIANA [7], can be integrated to facilitate semantic integration of prior knowledge in the model (see Chapter 7). At the core, intracellular, cellular, intercellular, and tissue-level scales can be integrated to model various spatiotemporal scales.

Table 8.1 Level of Multiscale Models and Their Properties		
Scale	Example Scenarios or Source	Spatiotemporal Scales
Summary of potential scales	Summary of published results	Semantic linkage between entities and scales
Intracellular	Signaling pathways	Millisecond, Nanometers
Cellular	Cell movement and subtypes	Seconds, Micrometers
Intercellular	Cytokine diffusion	Minutes, Millimeters
Tissue	Inflammation and lesions	Hours, Centimeters

Modeling Technologies and Tools

Although modeling technologies are diverse, current MSM tools take advantage of mainly equation-based and agent-based models (ABMs). Equation-based models are captured using mathematical equations, such as ODEs and PDEs. ODEs can easily capture entity changes in time but not in space. PDEs can capture changes in both time and space but are more complex to solve. In general, the complexity of equation-based models is determined by the number of equations describing the model. Mathematical equations are elegant and efficient representations; however, many biological phenomena cannot be easily captured using this mathematical formalism. In some instances, we do not fully understand the details of many of the biological phenomena to be able to represent them in mathematical equations; although in some cases assumptions can be made; however, depending on the biological process and the desirable predictive power of the model, these assumptions may not be sufficient for the mathematical formalism. Many biological systems are therefore modeled using ABMs. ABM comprised agents and their interactions. Like objects in objected-oriented (OO) design, agents in ABMs can capture arbitrary complex knowledge. For instance, agents can (i) have properties to represent different entity states, such as sex, genotypes, size, and color, (ii) be assigned to specific locations and move spatially, (iii) interact with the environment and other agents, and (iv) be represented in a hierarchical structure. ABM is capable of modeling multiscale and highly complex biological phenomena; furthermore, ABM can also integrate multiple modeling technologies.

Computational modeling technologies are highly intertwined with modeling tools and data. Furthermore, without user-friendly tools, modeling is a daunting task for scientists without adequate computational skills. As a result, a practical and valuable MSM tool will be judged not only based on the core quality of the model but also based on its user-friendliness and ability to assist biologically skilled scientists build useful multiscaled models to generate novel computational hypotheses. In fact, engineers can use Matlab to develop ODE-based models; however, computational biologists rely on tools such as COPASI [8] and Virtual Cell [9] due to their customized user-friendliness and usability features. COPASI provides user interfaces (UIs) for defining equations, entities, and rate laws (please refer to the Chapter 5 for further information about COPASI [10,11]). Biologically skilled scientists can utilize COPASI to model complex networks. For agent-based modeling, there are several existing tools such as SIMMUNE [12] and Basic Immune Simulator, BIS [13]; however, these are not designed to be easily extended to developing multiscale models of mucosal immune response. For generic modeling framework, computational biologists use NetLogo [14,15] or Repast [16]. NetLogo has better development efficiency while Repast provides enhanced flexibility, and Repast for high-performance computing (HPC) provides an added level of computational scalability.

From Single Scale to MSM

Computational modeling in biology dates back to 1970s [17], with earlier techniques that are based on reductionist approaches using mainly mathematical formalisms. However, with the emergence of computational technologies and introduction of computational systems, biology [18−20] and modeling techniques [21,22] have seen significant progress. For instance, equation-free modeling is being proposed for describing dynamic systems [23] as a result of a rapid increase in the computational power. In computational immunology, artificial immune systems [24,25] have emerged as an independent research area across multiple disciplines. Computational modeling techniques can capture existing knowledge into models and discover new knowledge through model analyses and simulations [2,25−28]. For instance, ODE models have been proposed for modeling the dynamics among HIV virus and immune cells [29], around the same time ABM with equation-based models were compared [30]. In fact, it is well accepted that ABM can be powerful tools [31] in computational biology. However, depending on the biological questions and available data, different techniques can be explored. Materi et al. [32] discussed computational modeling techniques, including ODE, PDE, and ABM, and tools used in drug discovery and development. At the software level, the virtual cell [9] provides an environment for modeling single cell using ODEs and PDEs.

One of the key challenges of MSM is the identification of appropriate linkages that facilitate integration of different computational models across scales. Hayenga et al. [33] argued that (i) vascular systems are complex and require faithful multiscale models composing of submodels at all scales (*macro, micro*, and *nano*) and (ii) efficiently coupling between submodels is critical for the performance of such models. Using Matlab, Krinner et al. [34] coupled an agent-based model of hematopoietic stem cells with an ODE model of granulopoiesis. More recently, Dwivedi et al. [35] presented a multiscale model, based on ODE, of interleukin-6—mediated immune regulation in Crohn's disease, one of the two main clinical manifestations of inflammatory bowel disease (IBD) and its application in drug discovery and development. An MSM approach was also utilized to identify the chemical, biological, and mechanical mechanisms of scar formation and wound healing where cross talk between these different fields (chemistry, biology, and mechanical engineering) could have a significant impact on wound management and individualized care [36]. The constitutive coupling between these fields was important for the general chemo-bio-mechanical problem. In the chemical fields, PDE was used for the reaction-diffusion systems; in the biological field, more complex PDE were designed that would account for variation in specialized cell population; and finally, the mechanical field was based on both PDE and ODE to model the mechanics of soft biological tissues [36]. Furthermore, novel software workflows are being developed for semantic integration of systems biology markup language (SBML)-based quantitative models in multiscaled tissue models and simulation [37]. For instance, by using EPISIM [37] or similar tools, it is possible to link cellular states such as differentiation to biochemical reaction networks. Furthermore, calibrated models can be integrated with a larger pool of existing models which are available in the Biomodels database [38]. Hence, over the past few decades, modeling and simulation efforts have moved from single small models of isolated biological system to a more comprehensive and integrated systems modeling approach that encompasses complex biological systems and human populations, where software have also been developed to aid biologically skilled scientists take advantage of modeling tools and generate

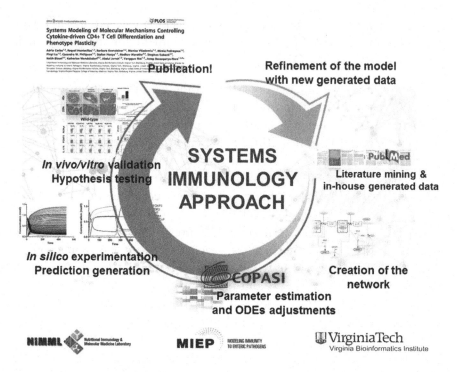

Figure 8.3 Iterative systems immunology perspective.

novel computational hypothesis that can be validated through preclinical or clinical trials (see Figure 8.3).

A broad array of simulators has been developed over the past decade to aid scientists in their modeling quests for discovering new knowledge. For instance, SIMMUNE [12] is a modeling environment that allows users to model and simulate cell–cell and cell–molecule interactions; it takes a generic approach and therefore can be used for a wide range of signaling cascades, including pathways that are directly related to immunology. ImmSim [39] is a very simple rule-based cellular automaton. However, due to the lack of modularity and scalability, the needed effort to refine and expand a generic simulator to a specific field is considerable and requires extensive technical knowledge. ImmSim was able to reproduce several phenomena in immunology. Basic Immune Simulator, BIS [13], and lymph node B-cell simulator [40] are two additional examples of immune simulators that are developed using open-source platforms. BIS was developed using Repast NetLogo [14,15], a popular ABM platform, and lymph node B-cell simulator was developed using Rhapsody [41]. They both provide suitable animations. Additional agent-based immune simulators include ParIMM [42], SIS [43], and NFSim [44]. Furthermore, Railsback et al. [45] surveyed several common platforms—Repast [16], Netlogo [14,15], and Swarm [46]—that could be used for the development of multiscale systems. Macal et al. [47] presented comparisons of the development approaches and concluded that in general, Netlogo and mathematic packages are easier to develop but provide less capabilities; Repast is more involved and complex but it provides added benefits and can be more powerful. Furthermore, Matlab is also widely used in computational modeling [34,48,49]. However, the latter is not open source. COPASI [8] is an open-source software tool that is based on C++ but provides language bindings to python and Java. COPASI is also SBML-compliant and provide practical UI for ODE-based models, it can therefore be used efficiently in the development of multiscale models that are modular and scalable. Hence, developing new MSM tools could be achieved by programming the software in Java, C++, or any other programming language and can be facilitated by adoption of common platforms. For instance, if an MSM tool uses function from Repast Symphony, it can be developed in Java but if the tool uses Repast HPC, then it can be developed in C++. However, a valuable tool is one that provides efficiency, modularity, and scalability in its internal structure but also a great visualization and refined UI.

SENSITIVITY ANALYSIS

SA is the study of the impact of different parameters on the outcomes of a system [50,51]. SA has been used in many scientific fields to highlight critical data, optimize the design of a system, simplify models, and rank the influence of various parameters on a given system [52−55]. In the context of MSM, SA can be very valuable in terms of model reduction, parameter estimation, and data analytics. For instance, reducing the number of parameters can significantly reduce the computational complexity of the model and allow more resources to be allocated towards generating larger *in silico* experimentations. Additionally, identification of important parameters can be fundamental towards our understanding of the systems dynamic and temporal behavior, which can lead to greater predictive power.

Developing novel SA methods for ABMs and ultimately multiscale models has the potential to improve the parameter estimation by making the process more systematic and streamlined. The objective of the SA is to identify the greatest and the least significant parameters of the model and to quantify how parameter uncertainty influences outcomes. However, analytical exploration of the behavior of complex systems is very challenging due to the large number of parameters and linear and nonlinear relationships among entities. On the other hand, system identification and reverse engineering methods can help to identify and understand the relationships between input and output variables; this understanding leads to appreciation of the robustness of the system and possibly identification of inaccuracies in the model.

SA can be performed at the global or local scale. Local SA examines the effect of deviations of parameters within its range, on system outcomes around a basal setting [56]. Global SA on the other hand, evaluates the entire parameter space to identify all of the system's critical points [52,57]. In the following section, local and global SA applied to ABMs are further defined and compared. More details on SA, especially applied to ABM can be found in Chapter 6. In the following sections, a summary is provided with emphasis on SA for multiscale models.

Global versus Local SA

In global SA, the focus is centered on the behavior of input parameters on the variation of the model output. In fact, different parameters have different (sometimes extreme) effect on the system's outcome. Given that some parameters play significant roles, while others are marginally important, make global SA a valuable tool. Local SA on the other hand measures the relative sensitivity of a single parameter value to changes in other parameters. Global SA requires higher computational power as compared to the local SA, and it is often supported by HPC systems.

A local SA addresses sensitivity relative to change of a single parameter value, while a global analysis examines sensitivity with regard to the entire parameter space. Global SA focuses on the variance of model outputs and determines how input parameters influence the output parameters. It is a quantitative and rigorous overview of how different inputs influence the output. Local SA focuses on a single input's behavior while other parts remain the same. The limitation of the local SA is in its limited scope, as the effect of input parameter is not measured for settings other than the basal level. For this reason, the global SA is often the preferred method; however, due to higher computational complexity, the global method may not always be the method of choice, in fact in many cases, local SA can be preferred.

Sparse Experimental Design for SA

Complex models of massively interacting systems such as the mucosal immune system with large parameter space require novel experimental design to address the computational costs of large-scale simulations. In fact, it is clear that not all possible combinations of parameter settings can be explored in this analysis. In a recent work, a novel design was proposed by our team to address this limitation [58]. The design strategy is based on an orthogonal array (OA) method [28,30,31]. A variation of this strategy has been widely used in many engineering applications [32] and SA of computer models [59]. An OA with strength t is a design matrix, such that for every column, the possible distinct rows all appear the same number of times. Such a property maintains the balance. More specification on this methodology can be found in Ref. [60]. In summary, this design strategy provides well-separated points in high-dimensional space to purposely limit the parameter space. This method is also further explained in Chapter 6.

Temporal Significance of Modeling Parameters

In any biological system, especially in more complex systems, different entities act or are acted upon at various level of specificity at different time during stress response to response to stimulus. Hence, studying the temporal significance of modeling parameters is important although it is often ignored due to complexity of the system. Interestingly, analyzing the temporal significance of parameters can help in reducing the parameter space based on the specific *in silico* study. For instance, in the model of *Helicobacter pylori* [27], Th1 and Th17 cell populations are at higher levels during the later stages of the infection, and therefore, the parameters associated with them have higher significance during the progression of the infection. In addition, it is possible to identify parameters that are critical for the transition to proinflammatory state. In the *H. pylori* study, the parameter responsible for the epithelial cell transitions to proinflammatory state (*Vec*) was identified to be critical to the response to *H. pylori*; in fact, *Vec* is an important parameter for the system as its increase translates to an increase in iTreg, Th1, Th17, M1, and M2 levels. Because this parameter is directly related to gut dysbiosis, its significance increases at chronic stages of the disease. Finally, to study the temporal significance of parameters, one must perform time course simulation studies with sufficient resolution. Evaluating the dynamic range of sensitive parameters will also be key in providing cues to reduction of parameter space. In essence, some parameters may have limited impact during the first stage of the infection, while others could be critical during the first stage and have limited weight during the final stages of the disease. Considering these subtle changes and quantifying these temporal behavior can have significant downstream effect on model calibration and computational hypothesis generation.

SA Across Scales

By using local and global sensitivity analyses, it is possible to identify the most significant parameters in the system. However, due to the complex nature of the massively interacting biological systems and the large parameter space, it is not possible to evaluate every system for every parameter combination. Expert knowledge and well-designed sparse frameworks are critical to address the computational challenges of parameter estimation and new SA methodologies.

In addition, multiscale models that integrate spatiotemporal scales spanning intracellular networks require more complex analysis; therefore performing SA across scales for such systems is even more challenging. These challenges arise from the lack of standards, large parameter space, and model complexity. In multiscale models, a model reduction approach that is based on the results of SA can lead to inaccuracies and poor models. Sensitive parameters that are key linkage between the scales are critical parameters; however, even less sensitive parameters that connect the scales are important and should not be discarded to reduce the model. For instance, cytokine inputs of the intracellular model depend on cytokine diffusion process at the tissue level, and tissue architecture depends on the cytokine production/degradation intracellularly. Cellular and intracellular models are interdependent with regard to phenotypic changes and cell—cell interactions occurring in the ABMs. The SA of multiscales models require careful evaluation especially if the results will be used for model reduction. Due to distinct spatiotemporal properties and computational performance requirements of different scales, model calibration and SA are best applied before model integration as well as following multiscale linkage can extend from inside the skin to outside the skin into human populations and *in silico* clinical trials.

Furthermore, because SA can be an effective tool for systematically identifying the most and the least significant parameters, it can provide valuable information on the robustness of the multiscale system if applied after model integration. In a systematic study, Wang et al. described an approach to achieve cross-scale SA that would link molecular signaling properties to cellular behavior [61]. Similarly, Summer et al., [62,63] proposed a different approach for the SA of multiscale models. The authors address SA of multiscale models by exploring group-based SA procedure, where SA is applied on groups of parameters. The result of this analysis can be used to identify the components of the model that are most important in determining the multiscale model behavior. The method was applied to a composite model of blood glucose homeostasis that combines models of processes at the subcellular, cellular, and organ level to describe the physiological system [62–64]. Finally, local as well as global sensitivity analyses should be performed whenever possible as a part of the modeling process. Global SA will quantify the sensitivity of the model due to parameter changes. Thus, it can be used to determine insignificant parameters for reducing the number of the parameters to be estimated during the fitting process. Local SA, performed following model calibration, will be used to determine the effect of the model on the parameters. A hybrid framework, similar to the SA framework described above, that uses sparse experimental design can also be valuable for large and more complex systems. The ultimate goal is to efficiently identify the most and the least significant parameters (or components) and unveils their contributions to the outcomes of the single or multiscale system. Results from SA can also be used for model reduction, parameter estimation, as well as analytics.

MSM OF MUCOSAL IMMUNE RESPONSES

Computational modeling tools and techniques are increasingly being applied to further advance a system-level mechanistic understanding of biological processes as well as to accelerate therapeutic development. Novel experimentations and innovative efforts are in part the product of *in silico* hypothesis generation. ENISI is an MSM tool for modeling the mucosal immune responses that can facilitate such knowledge discovery. During the development of ENISI [65], three versions were released; ENISI HPC [8] ENISI Visual [9], and ENISI MSM [10]. ENISI HPC focuses on scalability, ENISI Visual on visualizations, and ENISI MSM on the integration of heterogeneous modeling technologies.

The MSM framework has many valuable characteristics. For instance, we have shown that by implementing the system using Message Passing Interface (MPI) technology, it is possible to achieve great scalability for up to 576 processing elements when simulating 10 million cells [66,67]. In addition, the most recent version of the system, ENISI MSM [2], integrates COPASI, the ODE solver, ENISI, the agent-based simulator and ValueLayer library from Repast, and the PDE solver to model cytokine and chemokine diffusion. Furthermore, ENISI VISUAL has superior visualizations capabilities and empowers biologically skilled scientists to design and implement *in silico* experimentations with greater comfort and ease. More recently, we have developed an HPC-driven ENISI MSM (ENISI MSMv2) that integrates multiple technologies and is also able to scale to 10^9 agents on a cluster of 100 processors very efficiently (Table 8.2).

The Scales of ENISI Platform

Intracellular Scale: Intracellular scale models the signaling reactions at the protein level inside each individual cell during the immune response. ODE-based models, developed using COPASI [8], are used to represent the intracellular signaling pathways and transcriptional regulation. COPASI, a widely used ODE-based modeling tool in computational biology, was originally designed for biochemical reactions and was further expanded to model stochastic differential equations [6]. The three main steps for developing a COPASI model

Table 8.2 The Four Scales of ENISI Models, Their Spatial and Temporal Properties, As Well As Modeling Technologies and Tools for Each Scale

Scale	Example Scenarios	Spatial (m)	Time (s)	Technology	Tool
Intracellular	Signaling pathways	Nano	Nano	ODE	COPASI
Cellular	Cell movement and subtypes	Milli	Tens	ABM	ENISI
Intercellular	Cytokine diffusion	Milli	Tens	PDE	ValueLayer
Tissue	Inflammation and lesions	Centi	Thousands	Projections	ENISI

are (i) *developing the network model*, (ii) *calibrating the model*, and (iii) *performing analyses*. COPASI provides a simple UI for model development process.

Cellular Scale: ENISI simulates seven different immune cell types using ABMs. Each cell is an instance of an agent that has its own states and moves inside its designated compartments. Table 8.3 summarizes these different cell types and their states. The different immune cell types can have subtypes depending on the immune responses and their microenvironments.

Intercellular Scale: Cytokines and chemokines are secreted by cells and diffuse in the gut tissue microenvironment and are useful for engaging receptors on the cell surface and triggering signaling inside the cells. The cytokines, chemokines, and their change in concentration over time are modeled by PDE models. The PDE solver of ENISI

Table 8.3 Different Cell Types Modeled by ENteric Immune Simulator	
Cell Type	**Description**
Epithelial cells (Ep)	Organism's first line of defense. Intestinal Ep are continuously exposed to large numbers of commensal bacteria but are relatively insensitive to them. Following contact with pathogens, they produce inflammatory mediators and anti-microbial peptides
Macrophages (M)	Initiate the innate immune response against microbes. Depending on the environmental signals, macrophages can differentiate into at least two different subsets, M1 (proinflammatory) and M2 (anti-inflammatory)
Dendritic cells (DC)	Located at sites of pathogen entry in the gastrointestinal mucosa and involved in the induction of effector and regulatory responses. Immature DC have the capacity to internalize and process pathogens and present antigens via the MHC-class II pathway. Effector DC have a role in inducing T-cell-dependent effector responses such as T helper 1 (Th1) and Th17 responses. Tolerogenic DCs are a subset of DCs that mediate mechanisms of antigen specific tolerance induction in the periphery through induction of regulatory T cells (Treg)
Neutrophils (N)	Part of the innate immune system and highly motile. Neutrophils can be attracted by cytokines secreted by Ep and M and quickly move to the infected or inflamed areas. They can recruit and activate other immune cells, phagocyte pathogens, and release soluble antimicrobials
B cells	B cells are lymphocytes that play a major role in the humoral immune response. They produce antibodies against antigens, function as professional antigen-presenting cells, and eventually develop into memory B cells following activation by antigen interaction
T cells	CD4+ T cells are lymphocytes that mediate adaptive immune response. T cells usually are recruited by DCs and activate other immune cells such as B cells and M. Different phenotypes include T helper 1 (Th1), T helper 17 (Th17), and regulatory T cells (Treg)
Bacteria	Prokaryotic microorganisms; there are approximately ten times as many bacterial cells in the human flora as there are human cells in the body. The vast majority of the bacteria in the body are harmless, and some are even beneficial, for the immune and provide signals that facilitate tolerance and nutrition. However, a few species of bacteria are pathogenic and cause infectious diseases

Table 8.4 Compartments of the Immune System Modeled by ENteric Immune Simulator

Tissue Type	Description
Lumen	The inner open space of a tubular organ such as the stomach or intestine
Epithelium	The thin monolayer of epithelial cells separating the lumen and lamina propria
Lamina propria	The connective tissue underlying the epithelium where most of the immune cells associated with the stomach mucosa reside
Draining lymph nodes	The secondary lymphoid organs draining the gastrointestinal tract. The draining lymph nodes are inductive sites of the mucosal immune system
Blood	The source for the monocytes (e.g., macrophages, dendritic cells, and neutrophils)

MSM uses ValueLayer library of Repast [16], and the two main classes are GridValueLayer and ValueLayerDiffuser. GridVaueLayer stores the values for a grid space and provide methods to manipulate the values for individual grid cells. ValueLayerDiffuser diffuses the values of the GridValueLayer according to the two constants: evaporation constant and diffusion constant. The diffusion of cytokines and chemokines follows Eqn (8.1), where v_n is the value of the grid cell itself at step n. The values of c_e and c_d are evaporation constant and diffusion constant, respectively. The last part of the equation is the summation of the differences between all the neighboring cells and the cell itself.

$$v_n = c_e * \left[v_{n-1} + c_d * \sum \left(v_{n-1}^{neighbor} - v_{n-1} \right) \right], \qquad (8.1)$$

Tissue Scale: ENISI currently supports modeling five different tissue types, and these are implemented as compartment in two-dimensional spaces (see Table 8.4). The cells inside each tissue can be moved based on Brownian and chemokine-driven motions; these cells can also cross boundaries and move across different tissues. ENISI provides a practical UI that can be utilized to control the simulation settings (Figure 8.4). Further details regarding the visualization module, cellular and state transitions of ENISI can be found in Refs. [1,68].

Challenges and Opportunities

ENISI [65] is implemented in Java and based on the Repast Symphony [16], a reusable software architecture, and thus assures a level of robustness and integrity. COPASI is written in C++; however, it provides a Java language binding, which is instrumental in the development of this tool. The PDE solver library ValueLayer is part of Repast Symphony. The MSM tool that is based on the ENISI software

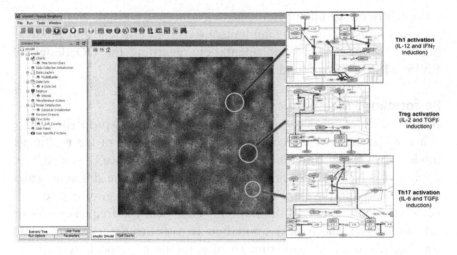

Figure 8.4 ENISI user interface. The left side is the control panels and users can set many simulation settings such as initial numbers of different cells, simulation speed, and ODE COPASI file path. The right side is the real-time simulation video with grids and icons of different colors. The regions highlighted correspond to Th1, Treg, as well as Th17 CD4+ T cell activation.

described thus far is being also implemented in C++ using the Repast HPC [69], which is written in C++ as well. This latest version of MSM technology provides greater scalability than current tools; it will be based on the next generation of ABM that is intended for large-scale distributed computing platforms. However, Repast HPC does not provide visualization capabilities similar to Repast Symphony. Other software (such as VisIt [70]) will be integrated with focus on visualization to complement the system. The ultimate goal is to have greater modeling capabilities with user-friendly interface. However, the hybrid modeling approach poses many challenges as well as many opportunities.

OO Design
ENISI MSM utilizes extensively OO programming features including encapsulations, inheritance, and polymorphism. In ENISI MSM cells, subcomponent (such as an ODE sub model) or cytokines with their propagation and dispersion following PDEs are represented by objects; in addition, many implementation details are encapsulated into objects. Furthermore, common data and methods are captured by a superclass that is inherited by multiple subclasses. In essence, the same method is implemented differently in the subclasses of different cell types to achieve polymorphism. The OO design is the only principle that can

consistently encapsulate heterogeneous concepts, entities, and relationship of multiscale models simultaneously in an efficient and modular manner. More detailed implementation regarding the OO design of ENISI MSM can be found in Refs. [1,2].

Performance Matching

Because different scales have different spatiotemporal properties, there is a need to increase the computational performance of the multiscale models by using different techniques. For instance, in a hybrid approach, ENISI MSM calls all the submodels in the different scales in each simulation cycle. For instance, if the simulation of one scale is performed once every 10 simulation cycles, then the frequency will be 0.1. In essence, the hybrid simulation frequencies across scales could significantly improve performance of a multiscale model. A different approach could be to limit the number of projections and the number of cytokines. However, the ODE solver COPASI object is still a large object, and therefore, loading millions of such objects in the memory could significantly slow the simulations. Alternatively, model reduction techniques can be valuable, where complex system can be reduced for MSM purposes. In addition, machine-learning methods (see Chapter 7) can also be used to estimate the system's behavior in exchange for higher computational power. Multiscale model development may require modifying the single layer submodels before coupling them together into a multiscale model. The reduction in model complexity and loss in accuracy can be compensated with higher computational power for model simulations and more realistic number of agents for *in silico* studies.

HPC-Driven MSM of Mucosal Immune Responses

ENISI MSMv2 is the latest version of the MSM technology that we have developed. The system is based on REPAST for HPC. REPAST for HPC [69] is intended for large-scale distributed computing platforms and implements the core Repast Simphony [16] concepts. REPAST HPC, written in cross-platform C++ language, is also an open source but modified to work in parallel distributed environment. In addition, REPAST HPC uses MPI for distributed processing. The framework provides a useful and usable working system. Repast HPC is maintained and tested by Argonne National Laboratory and provides a useful and usable working system for the implementation of ABMs. However, the framework is not as well documented as

REPAST Simphony and does not have all the key functionalities, such as visualization module, and a comprehensive ValueLayer library. Using the model described above, ENISI MSMv2 is used to model the gut inflammation by using the CD4+ T-cell differentiation ODE model and connecting specific molecular events occurring inside the cell with major changes at the tissue level, such as changes of tissue architecture and immunopathologies occurring at the cellular and tissue levels. The multiscale model developed clearly demonstrates the capabilities of the system as a user-friendly MSM platform, specifically aimed for higher resolution and larger modeling studies. REPAST HPC is intended for large-scale distributed computing and can greatly improve the performance of the MSM tool. The transition from REPAST Simphony to REPAST HPC is an important step that required further development of the core system and is currently being optimized for distributed computing and large *in silico* experimentation from 10^9 to 10^{12} agents. Finally, as shown, larger simulations studies clearly enhance the predictive power for *in silico* experimentation (see Case Study).

Future of MSM

ENISI is the first MSM platform for modeling mucosal immune responses. ENISI MSM has modular, coherent, and user-friendly UI, and superior visualization. ENISI can accelerate the development of comprehensive multiscale models of massively interacting systems by computational immunologists and therefore maintains and supports the *in silico* experimentation process for model-driven computational hypothesis generation. Using an OO design and integrating different scales and different technologies systematically highlights the computational power of the system. In addition, such system is well aligned with the field of integrative systems biology and can greatly enhance our modeling practices in general. ENISI MSMv2 is at the cutting edge of MSM of the mucosal immune responses (in preparation). ENISI MSMv2 is currently being further optimized to scale to unprecedented levels of complexity. The tool integrates different spatiotemporal scales and different technologies while performing large-scale *in silico* experimentation that are able to scale to 10^9 and beyond.

In conclusion, a plethora of computational tools has been developed in recent years to address the need of the scientific community [12,13,32,39,40,42,44]; however, the challenges of modeling and in particular MSM framework are diverse and multilateral. ENISI's modeling environment addresses some of these challenges by adopting an integrated OO design principle. In addition, we are actively working towards further addressing these challenges by implementing the system using HPC. HPC-driven ENISI MSM enhances development of massively interacting models of the mucosal immune system and significantly increase the power of the *in silico* experimentation (i.e., modeling systems with $>10^{10}$ agents). The state-of-the-art technologies will be instrumental in the development of a scalable system. Furthermore, as previously demonstrated [71−73], artificial neural networks as well as Random Forest algorithms are efficient alternatives to ODEs and can reduce the complexity of intracellular network models. Integration of Machine Learning methodology for well-documented signaling pathways can also significantly increase scalability and performance for larger networks. Finally, further enhancing the visualization component of the system can directly enhance its adoption by experimentalists. Work is in the pipeline to make the platform interoperable with VisIt [70]. In summary, ENISI empowers the immunology community to accelerate the fast and cost-effective knowledge discovery.

CASE STUDY

Modeling Mucosal Immunity in the Gut

In this section, two multiscale models are described. These models can be used to run *in silico* simulations and generate computational hypothesis for further experimental validation. These models can also be used to test an array of hypothetical scenarios that are not possible to analyze with single-scale models; thus linking specific molecular events occurring inside the cell with major changes at the tissue level, such as changes of tissue architecture and immunopathologies occurring at the cellular and tissue levels. The multiscale model developed demonstrates the capabilities of ENISI MSM as an MSM platform in the field of immunology.

Multiscale Model for IBD

A multiscale model of gut inflammation developed using the ENISI MSM system is presented to demonstrate the stages of MSM in a practical setting. The IBD multiscale model is based on three submodels (ABM, ODE, and PDE) to represent the different scales.

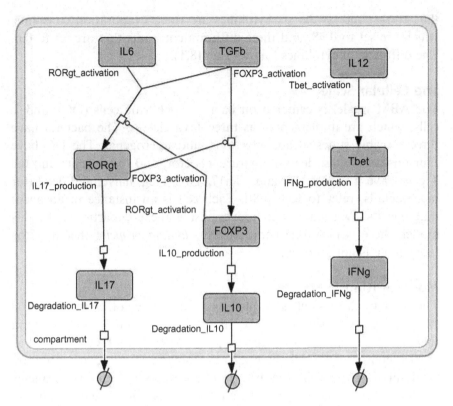

Figure 8.5 The network of simplified CD4+ T-cell differential model utilized for the development of the ODE model.

The Intracellular Scale

The ODE model that is implemented in COPASI, is a simplified version of the comprehensive CD4+ T-cell differentiation model [26,74,75]. The network of the model (Figure 8.5) can be developed in CellDesigner and imported into COPASI. This model is based on six cytokines, three as inputs and three as outputs. The three input cytokines are IL-12, TGFβ, and IL-6. The three output cytokines are INFγ, IL-17, and IL-10. The COPASI ODE solver has a main object CCopasiDataModel that can load a COPASI model file for the initialization process.

The Intercellular Scale

The ODE solver class also provides a hashMap for storing the concentrations of cytokines and chemokines. Those concentrations provide the initial values for entities in the model. The six ValueLayer objects that correspond to the six cytokines are three evaporation constants, which are set to 0.98, and three diffusion constants that are set to 0.6. The diffusion of cytokines follows Eqn (8.1).

The Cellular Scale

The ABM model is centered on bacteria, dendritic cells (DC), and T cells, which are implemented as three Java classes. The bacteria have three possible states: dead, infectious, and tolerogenic. The DC have four possible states: dead, immature, effector, and tolerogenic; and the T cells have five possible states: Th17, Th1, Treg, naive, and dead (for more details, refer to Ref. [68]). Each cell is an instance of an agent that has its own states and moves inside the compartment. In this model, there is only one compartment, *lamina propria*, therefore the tissue scale is not modeled.

Model Settings

The area in the model is defined as a square region with 100×100 two-dimensional grid cells. The simulation stats with 1000 bacteria (half infectious and half tolerogenic) and 2000 naive T cells as well as 2000 immature DC. All these agents (bacteria, T cells, and DC) are randomly distributed in the grid. In one simulation cycle, these agents can move to any direction with an evenly distributed speed that can range between zero and one grid cell side length. During the simulation, when agents are initialized and subsequently move, different scenarios can arise. (1) since agents are randomly distributed in the grid, some regions can have tolerogenic DC and some regions effector DC; furthermore, since cytokines are diffusing and evaporating, some regions will have only TGF-β and some other regions will have TGFβ and IL-6. Therefore, naive T cells will differentiate into the different subtypes (or states) such as Treg, Th17, or Th1 cells depending on their location and the cytokines present in those regions. Given the input concentrations of cytokines, the ODE model will perform the time course simulation and calculate the output cytokines concentrations (IFNγ, IL-17, and IL-10) that will be released in the microenvironment. (2) The immature DC can become in contact with the infectious or tolerogenic bacteria (in the same grid). In the first situation, the iDC will differentiate into effector subtype and the effector DC will release IL-6 and Il-12 into the tissue microenvironment, by setting the concentrations of the two cytokine value layer to a relative value (in this case 70) at that grid cell. In the second situation, the iDC will differentiate into tolerogenic dendritic cells (tDCs) and release TGF-β into the tissue microenvironment.

Simulation

During each simulation cycle, the quantitative information (such as cell count) can be visualized. The grid cell background color is visualized based on the cytokine concentrations; the three cytokines are visualized as three primary colors. The color codes are designed to represent in red regions with higher Th1, in purple regions with higher Th17, and in blue regions with higher Treg cells. Furthermore, the intracellular ODE simulation results are displayed as texts in the terminal window for visual inspection during the simulation; the latter could be saved for further analysis.

ENISI MSM incorporates a stochastic component that leads to differential concentration level of various agents. For instance, in some regions, there will be higher concentration of Th1, while in other regions, the concentration of Th17 cells can be higher. In addition, since the cell count can be viewed over time for the different species, it will highlight the temporal evolution of the immune response and the concentration of the different cell types over the course of the simulation. As an example in this study, the concentration of Th1, Th17, and Treg cell subsets are increasing in the initial stage of the simulation; however, after about 20 cycles, Th17 is the dominant cell type [1]. This trend is due to the fact that the cytokines were isolated during the initial stage, and changes were made during the diffusion process and the inter-association and transformation of the agents in the later stages. As we will show, this artifact will disappear with larger *in silico* experimentation using ENISI MSMv2.

As a proof of concept, a multiscale model of gut inflammation was also developed using the ENISI MSMv2. Interesting observations, from the *in silico* experimentation are the dynamics and temporal behavior of the various cell types during inflammation. For instance, as the naive T cells are differentiated into various subtypes, there is a clear distinction between the production rate of regulatory and anti-inflammatory cell types (Figure 8.6). This dynamics is different from models that were developed with very limited number of agents using the ENISI MSM prototype implemented in REPAST Simphony. In the previous *in silico* model [2], where 5000 agents were used, the

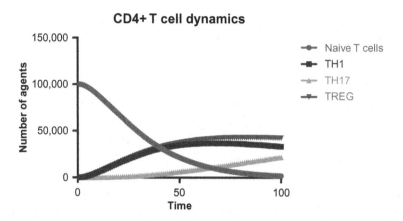

Figure 8.6 Average number of CD4+ T-cell subtypes during gut inflammation. Simulation is performed using ENISI MSMv2 using a total of 250,000 agents. Source: Data from simulation study is streamlined and visualized in VisIt.

production of Th17 cells clearly dominated the other cell types; however, in this model, there is a balance. The T-cell dynamics illustrated in this model is more relevant immunologically and consistent with what would be expected during gut inflammation associated with immune-mediated disease such as Crohn's disease. We are working on further simulation studies to better understand the nature of this temporal characteristic as well as the underlying cytokine combinations that allow this outcome.

MSM of Mucosal Immune Responses

Given the complexity of the interaction of *H. pylori* with the human gastric mucosa, the use of multiscale models can aid in the elucidation of the cellular and molecular mechanisms that determine the outcome of the infection. For instance, *H. pylori* induce a mixed CD4+ T cell response characterized by the presence of cells with Th17, Th1, and Treg functions. Induction of Treg has been linked to more effective colonization, while Th17 is associated with suppressed bacterial burden [76]. Our ODE model of *H. pylori* infection has revealed that the interaction between epithelial cells and macrophages might be critical for the pathological output. Moreover, macrophage phenotype was shown to also modulate the levels of bacterial colonization [27]. MSM can be used to integrate and synthesize data sets across all the elements participating in the response to *H. pylori*. Using the ENISI MSM system, a multiscale model calibrated with experimental data can be constructed

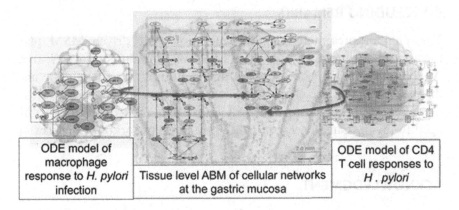

| ODE model of macrophage response to *H. pylori* infection | Tissue level ABM of cellular networks at the gastric mucosa | ODE model of CD4 T cell responses to *H . pylori* |

Figure 8.7 Schematic representation of the strategy for the development a multiscale model of the gastric mucosa immune responses to H. pylori *integrating single-cell ODE models of the cell types of interest.*

based on three submodels (ABM, ODE, and PDE) to represent the different scales. The computational model of the immune response to *H. pylori* [27] (see Chapter 3) can be further refined based on novel experimental findings. For instance, the tissue-level agent-based model of cellular networks at the gastric mucosa can be expanded by the integration of an internal ODE-based models representing perturbations on macrophages [77] and CD4+ T cells in response to *H. pylori* [26,75] (see Figure 8.7). Other than increasing the granularity of the system by allowing a detailed evaluation of the events taking place in each specific cell type, the multiscale model can also serve to integrate different data types, including high throughput single-cell flow cytometry data or time series RNA-Seq with stomach bacterial loads following infection. The ABM model is also further calibrated and analyzed using various techniques such as global and local SA. In this way, one can address scientific questions such as how a transcription factor altered in macrophages following *H. pylori* infection affects the balance of effector versus regulatory responses in CD4+ T cells and the consequences in bacterial levels and lesion development. The MSM approach allow our team to investigate key questions by integrating deterministic as well as rule-based models to represents mechanistic models of *H. pylori*.

While the first case study provided a detailed modeling approach, the second case study provides a view of a more complex multiscale model and the opportunities of knowledge discovery that could be driven by multilevel analytics and *in silico* experimentation. MSM can clearly expedite the research outcome by providing novel directions for experimentations.

CONCLUDING REMARKS

This chapter presented the next-generation HPC-driven MSM platforms and technologies with the focus on immunological research. Analytics, such as SA across scales and performance matching are also discussed. Finally, the chapter ends with two case studies related to the modeling of the mucosal immunity in the gut. The reader is encouraged to review Chapter 9 for further step-by-step workout examples.

ACKNOWLEDGMENT

This work was supported in part by National Institute of Allergy and Infectious Diseases Contract No. HHSN272201000056C to J. Bassaganya-Riera and funds from the Nutritional Immunology and Molecular Medicine Laboratory (www.nimml.org).

REFERENCES

[1] Mei Y, et al. Multiscale modeling of mucosal immune responses. BMC Bioinformatics 2015; 16 Suppl 12:S2.

[2] Mei Y, et al. ENISI MSM: a novel multi-scale modeling platform for computational immunology. In: 2014 IEEE International Conference on Bioinformatics and Biomedicine. 2014. p. 391–396.

[3] Le Novere N. Quantitative and logic modelling of molecular and gene networks. Nat Rev Genet 2015;16(3):146–58.

[4] Zou M, Conzen SD. A new dynamic Bayesian network (DBN) approach for identifying gene regulatory networks from time course microarray data. Bioinformatics 2005;21 (1):71–9.

[5] Punta M, Simon I, Dosztányi Z. Prediction and analysis of intrinsically disordered proteins. In: Owens RJ, editor. Structural proteomics. New York: Springer; 2015. p. 35–59.

[6] Mei YG, et al. ENISI SDE: a novel web-based stochastic modeling tool for computational biology. 2013 IEEE International Conference on Bioinformatics and Biomedicine (Bibm). 2013.

[7] Abedi V, Yeasin M, Zand R. Empirical study using network of semantically related associations in bridging the knowledge gap. J Transl Med 2014;12:324.

[8] Hoops S, et al. COPASI—a COmplex PAthway SImulator. Bioinformatics 2006;22 (24):3067–74.

[9] Loew LM, Schaff JC. The Virtual Cell: a software environment for computational cell biology. Trends Biotechnol 2001;19(10):401–6.

[10] MIEP. Modeling Immunity to Entering Pathogens. COPSAI SUITE; 2015. Available from: http://www.modelingimmunity.org/tools/copasi-suite.

[11] Mendes P, et al. Computational modeling of biochemical networks using COPASI. In: Maly IV, editor. Systems biology. Humana Press; 2009. p. 17–59.

[12] Meier-Schellersheim M. SIMMUNE, a tool for simulating and analyzing immune system behavior. Hamburg: University of Hamburg; 1999.

[13] Folcik VA, An GC, Orosz CG. The Basic Immune Simulator: an agent-based model to study the interactions between innate and adaptive immunity. Theor Biol Med Model 2007;4:39.

[14] Sklar E. NetLogo, a multi-agent simulation environment. Artif Life 2007;13(3):303−11.

[15] Tisue S, Wilensky U. Netlogo: a simple environment for modeling complexity. In: International Conference on Complex Systems. 2004. p. 16−21.

[16] Collier N, Howe TR, North MJ. Onward and upward: the transition to Repast 2.0. Proceedings of the first annual North American Association for Computational Social and Organizational Science Conference. Pittsburgh: Carnegie Mellon University; 2003.

[17] DeLisi C. Mathematical modeling in immunology. Annu Rev Biophys Bioeng 1983;12:117−38.

[18] Kitano H. Computational systems biology. Nature 2002;420(6912):206−10.

[19] Hucka M, et al. The systems biology markup language (SBML): a medium for representation and exchange of biochemical network models. Bioinformatics 2003;19(4):524−31.

[20] Davison DB, et al. Whither computational biology. J Comput Biol 1994;1(1):1−2.

[21] Brown CT, et al. New computational approaches for analysis of cis-regulatory networks. Dev Biol 2002;246(1):86−102.

[22] Yuh CH, Bolouri H, Davidson EH. Genomic cis-regulatory logic: experimental and computational analysis of a sea urchin gene. Science 1998;279(5358):1896−902.

[23] Ye H, et al. Equation-free mechanistic ecosystem forecasting using empirical dynamic modeling. Proc Natl Acad Sci USA 2015;112(13):E1569−76.

[24] Klarreich E. Inspired by immunity. Nature 2002;415(6871):468−70.

[25] Forrest S, Beauchemin C. Computer immunology. Immunol Rev 2007;216:176−97.

[26] Carbo A, et al. Systems modeling of molecular mechanisms controlling cytokine-driven CD4+ T cell differentiation and phenotype plasticity. PLoS Comput Biol 2013;9(4): e1003027.

[27] Carbo A, et al. Predictive computational modeling of the mucosal immune responses during Helicobacter pylori infection. PLoS One 2013;8(9):e73365.

[28] Grimm V, et al. Pattern-oriented modeling of agent-based complex systems: lessons from ecology. Science 2005;310(5750):987−91.

[29] Perelson A, Nelson P. Mathematical analysis of HIV-1 dyamics *in vivo*. SIAM Rev 1999; 41(1):3−44.

[30] Parunak HV, Savit R, Riolo RL. Agent-based modeling vs. equation-based modeling: a case study and users' guide. Multi Agent Syst Agent Based Simul 1998;1534:10−25.

[31] Macal C, North M. Tutorial on agent-based modeling and simulation. J Simul 2010;8 (2):177−83.

[32] Materi W, Wishart DS. Computational systems biology in drug discovery and development: methods and applications. Drug Discov Today 2007;12(7−8):295−303.

[33] Hayenga H, et al. Multiscale computational modeling in vascular biology: from molecular mechanisms to tissue-level structure and function. In: Amit G, editor. Multiscale computer modeling in biomechanics and biomedical engineering. Berlin Heidelberg: Springer; 2013. p. 209−40.

[34] Krinner A, et al. Merging concepts—coupling an agent-based model of hematopoietic stem cells with an ODE model of granulopoiesis. BMC Syst Biol 2013;7:117.

[35] Dwivedi G, et al. A multiscale model of interleukin-6-mediated immune regulation in Crohn's disease and its application in drug discovery and development. CPT Pharmacometrics Syst Pharmacol 2014;3:e89.

[36] Buganza Tepole A, Kuhl E. Computational modeling of chemo-bio-mechanical coupling: a systems-biology approach toward wound healing. Comput Methods Biomech Biomed Engin 2014:1–18.

[37] Sutterlin T, et al. Bridging the scales: semantic integration of quantitative SBML in graphical multi-cellular models and simulations with EPISIM and COPASI. Bioinformatics 2013;29(2):223–9.

[38] Mc Auley MT, et al. Nutrition research and the impact of computational systems biology. J Comput Sci Syst Biol 2013;6(5):271–85.

[39] Puzone R, et al. IMMSIM, a flexible model for in machina experiments on immune system responses. Future Generation Comput Syst 2002;18(7):961–72.

[40] Swerdlin N, Cohen IR, Harel D. The lymph node B cell immune response: dynamic analysis in-silico. Proc IEEE 2008;96(8):1421–43.

[41] Gery E, Harel H, Palachi E. Rhapsody: a complete life-cycle model-based development system. In: Butler M, Petre L, Sere K, editors. Integrated formal methods. Berlin Heidelberg: Springer; 2002. p. 1–10.

[42] Bernaschi M, Castiglione F. Design and implementation of an immune system simulator. Comput Biol Med 2001;31(5):303–31.

[43] Mata J, Cohn M. Cellular automata-based modeling program: synthetic immune system. Immunol Rev 2007;216:198–212.

[44] Sneddon MW, Faeder JR, Emonet T. Efficient modeling, simulation and coarse-graining of biological complexity with NFsim. Nat Methods 2011;8(2):177–83.

[45] Railsback S, Lytinen S, Jackson S. Agent-based simulation platforms: review and development recommendations. Simulation 2006;82(9):609–23.

[46] Swarm. Available from: http://www.swarm.org. 2015.

[47] Macal C, North M. Introduction to agent-based modeling and simulation. Argonne, IL: Argonne National Laboratory; 2006.

[48] Keating SM, et al. SBML Toolbox: an SBML toolbox for MATLAB users. Bioinformatics 2006;22(10):1275–7.

[49] Weaver DC, Workman CT, Stormo GD. Modeling regulatory networks with weight matrices. Pac Symp Biocomput 1999;4:112–23.

[50] Saltelli A, et al. Variance based sensitivity analysis of model output. Design and estimator for the total sensitivity index. Comput Phys Commun 2010;181(2):259–70.

[51] Helton J. Uncertainty and sensitivity analysis for models of complex systems. In: Graziani F, editor. Computational methods in transport: verification and validation. Berlin Heidelberg: Springer; 2008. p. 207–28.

[52] Cacuci D, Ionescu-Bujor M, Navon I. Sensitivity and uncertainty analysis: applications to large-scale systems, vol. ii. New York: Chapman & Hall/CRC; 2005.

[53] Brooks R, Semenov M, Jamieson P. Simplifying Sirius: sensitivity analysis and development of a meta-model for wheat yield prediction. Eur J Agron 2001;14(1):43–60.

[54] Do H, Rothermel G. Using sensitivity analysis to create simplified economic models for regression testing. Proceedings of the 2008 International Symposium on Software Testing and Analysis. Seattle, WA: ACM; 2008. p. 51–62.

[55] Sher AA, et al. A local sensitivity analysis method for developing biological models with identifiable parameters: application to cardiac ionic channel modelling. Future Generation Comput Syst 2013;29(2):591–8.

[56] Frey H, Patil S. Identification and review of sensitivity analysis methods. Risk Anal 2002;22(3):553–78.

[57] Hamby D. A comparison of sensitivity analysis techniques. Health Phys 1995;68 (2):195–204.

[58] Alam M, et al. Sensitivity analysis of an ENteric Immunity SImulator (ENISI)-based model of immune responses to *Helicobacter pylori* infection. PloS one 2015;10:e0136139.

[59] Morris M, Moore L, McKay M. Using orthogonal arrays in the sensitivity analysis of computer models. Technometrics 2008;50(2):205–15.

[60] Hedayat A, Sloane N, Stufken J. Orthogonal arrays: theory and applications. New York: Springer; 1999. p. 417.

[61] Wang Z, Birch CM, Deisboeck TS. Cross-scale sensitivity analysis of a non-small cell lung cancer model: linking molecular signaling properties to cellular behavior. Biosystems 2008;92(3):249–58.

[62] Sumner T, et al. A composite computational model of liver glucose homeostasis. II. Exploring system behaviour. J R Soc Interface 2012;9(69):701–6.

[63] Sumner T, Shephard E, Bogle ID. A methodology for global-sensitivity analysis of time-dependent outputs in systems biology modelling. J R Soc Interface 2012;9(74):2156–66.

[64] Summer T. Sensitivity analysis in systems biology modelling and its application to a multiscale model of blood glucose homeostasis. Centre for Mathematics and Physics in the Life Sciences and Experimental Biology. London: University College; 2010. p. 162.

[65] MIEP. Modeling Immunity to Entering Pathogens. ENISI SUITE; 2015; Available from: http://www.modelingimmunity.org/tools/enisi-suite.

[66] Bisset K, et al. High-performance interaction-based simulation of gut immunopathologies with ENteric Immunity SImulator (ENISI). 2012 IEEE 26th International Parallel and Distributed Processing Symposium (IPDPS); 2012. p. 48–59.

[67] Wendelsdorf K, et al. ENteric Immunity SImulator: a tool for *in silico* study of gastroenteric infections. IEEE Trans NanoBioScience 2012;11:273–88.

[68] Mei Y, et al. ENISI Visual, an agent-based simulator for modeling gut immunity. IEEE International Conference of Bioinformatics and Biomedicine (BIBM); 2012.

[69] Collier N, North M. Repast HPC: a platform for large-scale agent-based modeling. Large-scale computing. John Wiley & Sons, Inc.; 2012. p. 81–109.

[70] Childs H, et al. VisIt: an end-user tool for visualizing and analyzing very large data. In: Wes Bethel E, Childs H, Hansen C, editors. High performance visualization, enabling extreme-scale scientific insight. FL: CRC Press; Boca Raton; 2012. p. 357–72.

[71] Lu P, et al. Suervised learning methods in modeling of CD4+ T cell heterogeneity. BioData Min 2015;8:27.

[72] Lu P, et al. Supervised learning with artificial neural networks in modeling of cell differentiation processes. Emerging trends in computational biology, bioinformatics and systems biology. Burlignton, MA: Morgan Kaufmann; 2015.

[73] Mei Y, et al. Neural network models for classifying immune cell subsets. In: BIBM. Shanghai, China; 2013.

[74] Carbo A, et al. Systems modeling of the role of interleukin-21 in the maintenance of effector CD4+ T cell responses during chronic *Helicobacter pylori* infection. MBio 2014;5(4): e01243-14

[75] Carbo A, et al. Computational modeling of heterogeneity and function of CD4+ T cells. Front Cell Dev Biol 2014;2:31.

[76] Ding H, et al. Th1-mediated immunity against *Helicobacter pylori* can compensate for lack of Th17 cells and can protect mice in the absence of immunization. PLoS One 2013;8(7):e69384.

[77] Philipson CW, et al. Modeling the Regulatory Mechanisms by which NLRX1 Modulates Innate Immune Responses to Helicobacter pylori infection. PLos One 2015.

CHAPTER *9*

Modeling Exercises

Vida Abedi[1], Stefan Hoops[1], Raquel Hontecillas[1], Adria Carbo[2], Casandra Philipson[2], Monica Viladomiu[1], Andrew Leber[1], Pinyi Lu[1], and Josep Bassaganya-Riera[1]

[1]Nutritional Immunology and Molecular Medicine Laboratory, Virginia Bioinformatics Institute, Virginia Tech, Blacksburg, VA, USA [2]Biotherapeutics Inc., Blacksburg, VA, USA

MODELING TOOLS

A key feature of a practical and valuable modeling tool rests in its ability to assist biologically-skilled scientists build useful models to generate novel hypotheses. Engineers can use Matlab to develop ordinary differential equation (ODE)−based models; however, computational biologists rely on tools such as the COmplex PAthway SImulator (COPASI) [1] to model complex networks. There are also tools that are specifically designed for agent based as well as multiscaled modeling, including SIMMUNE [2] and Basic Immune Simulator, BIS [3], and more recently the ENISI suite [4−6]; however, many of these are not tailored to be easily extended for developing models of enteric immune systems. For generic modeling framework, computational biologists can also use NetLogo [7,8] or Repast [9]. NetLogo has better development efficiency while Repast provides better flexibility and performance. Moreover, the high-performance computing capability of Repast provides greater scalability feature.

COPASI [1] is an open-source software tool that is based on C++ but provides language bindings to python and Java; it is SBML-compliant and provide practical user interface (UI) for ODE-based models. COPASI can also be used efficiently in the development of multiscale models that are modular and scalable. COPASI provide UIs for defining equations, entities, and rate laws and is specifically designed to target biologically skilled scientists with limited knowledge of mathematical equations for modeling complex networks. COPASI

Computational Immunology: Models and Tools. DOI: http://dx.doi.org/10.1016/B978-0-12-803697-6.00009-6

currently supports only ODE-based models. The tool is widely used for modeling "inside the cell" signaling/transcriptional networks inside the cell and performing steady state and time course analyses. In addition, all the ODE reactions in COPASI are first order, and users can specify the rate of such reactions and change the parameters in the rate functions. COPASI was further expanded to model stochastic differential equations [5]. The three main steps for developing a COPASI model are summarized here:

> Developing the network model: Development of the model topology, which does not include dynamical properties, can be achieved using CellDesigner [10]. The initial model can then be imported into COPASI where additions can be made to the model. For instance, dynamical specifications can be added to all the ODEs for all the reactions.
>
> Calibrating the model: Model calibration focuses on parameter estimation by fitting the simulations generated by the model with experimental data, extracted from the literature or directly from wet-lab. COPASI provides UI for the model calibration process.
>
> Performing analyses: The types of analyses that can be performed in COPASI include metabolic, steady state, time course, and sensitivity analyses, etc.

In the following section, we will demonstrate how these steps can be taken to develop and calibrate a model and perform analysis to generate new model-based hypothesis. We will demonstrate these examples using the tools, COPASI and CellDesigner, commonly used by computational biologists.

MODELS

Computational Model of Immune Responses to *Clostridium difficile* Infection

As the first step in building a computational model of *C. difficile*, we will construct a general network that is based on an initial experimental findings or published literature. The network at this stage often comprised known interactions, which will give the model a strong foundation for future expansion and experimentation. Furthermore, the model building process is iterative; hence, the network model constructed at this stage will evolve throughout the modeling process.

The network used in this example, the immune responses to *C. difficile* model, was constructed to include multiple layers within the colon and associated immune system. The network is built to analyze the changes that occur on a cellular level. However, the model can also be used in a multiscale setting.

It is important, at an initial step, to focus on a single biological scale (molecular, cellular, etc.) when building the network. When constructing your own model, you will likely already have a good understanding of the related literature; however, it is still important to scan the literature in order to identify recent findings. For instance, in the *C. difficile* example, PubMed was used to further support the five activation interactions (see the associations in Figure 9.1 in bold). It is important to use only general terms during the research process (e.g., "*C. difficile*," "cellular response," "host immunity," or "inflammatory response"). All types of studies are useful during this stage. Clinical and *in vivo* studies can serve to show the importance and impact of a factor on the overall system in a realistic setting. Meanwhile, *in vitro*

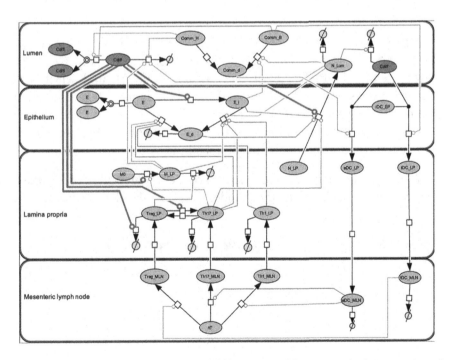

Figure 9.1 The network model of C. difficile. *The model was generated from an extensive literature review and experimental data and implemented into network form in the program CellDesigner.*

studies help to focus in on a particular interaction and can help to confirm direct links between species. It is important to be flexible at this stage, and fine-tuning of the network can be done during the later stages of model development.

Creating the model in CellDesigner: To create a model in CellDesigner go to *File → New*, then Enter a *name* and *size* of the model and then *Select OK*.

There are different options in the toolbar that you can use. *Species*: Different shapes designed to represent protein, simple molecules, receptors, genes, and more. Choose coloring options or shapes to populate different species of the model. *Reaction*: Connections with arrows are used to mark a state transition of a cell, association of a complex, or a chemical reaction. Connections that end in a circle or perpendicular line connect a species to a transition and are typically used for activators or inhibitors. The properties of species (such as name, color, and size) can be modified by right clicking on the object.

Finally, you can now *Save* the model in CellDesigner as an .xml or .sbml file.

Importing the model in COPASI (see Figure 9.2): You can import the model that was developed in CellDesigner directly into COPASI. After opening COPASI, select *File → Import* SBML and select your file. All species or nodes that created in CellDesigner will be entered as species. Transition interactions, represented by arrows in CellDesigner will be assigned to reactions. Activation and inhibition interactions will be imported as modifiers to the reactions.

Defining reactions in COPASI: To view the reactions, expand the reactions section in the model tree in the left pane of the

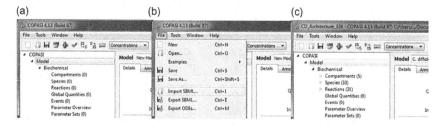

Figure 9.2 *Importing the model into COPASI. (a) COPASI prior to model import. (b) Import SBML file. (c) COPASI after model import.*

COPASI window. Reactions that are described in terms of reactants, products, and modifiers have to be defined by equations. After clicking on a particular reaction, you can view the suggested rate laws from COPASI's function bank in the dropdown menu next to rate law. Most often, it is best to start simple with the rate laws and attempt to work with the model and adjust complexity to address problems or issues that arise. Therefore, to begin assigning rate laws, mass action and simple activation–inhibition laws should be selected. *Mass action rate laws* are particularly relevant for degradation or death reactions and often sufficiently function in this capacity even for final models. If the activation or inhibition requires a more complex method of implementation, a *Michaelis–Menten*-like of *Hill-type reaction* can be used. If the network contains multiple modifiers per reactions, COPASI may not have an exact match for your desired rate law. However, the functions provided by COPASI will often give you an outline for how to implement a new rate law. Additionally, when working with multiple modifiers, it is often best to add separate terms for each modifier. For instance, two activators in simple activation is likely better represented by k1*S*A1 + k2*S*A2 rather than k*S*A1*A2.

Choose a reaction and assign a rate law from the dropdown box. Try to minimize the number of parameters that are needed for each reaction. If the reaction contained one or more modifiers, ensure that they appear in the mapping column. The items that appear in the "Symbol Definition" box are color-coded (red: substrate, green: product, blue: parameter, and yellow: modifier). Alternatively, you can enter your own rate laws by clicking "New Rate Law." The formula that will be written will be set to be negative in the differential equation describing the rate of change of the substrate in the given reaction and positive in the differential equation describing the rate of change of the product. After writing the formula, click the button in the upper right that appears as the square root of x to implement the formula. Additionally, you will need to assign a description for each variable in the formula in the "Parameters" box in the lower half of the panel. Choose the correct description from the dropdown menu. After creating the rate law, you can go back to the reaction and select it from the dropdown menu. Also, reactions can be reversible or irreversible (e.g., reversible reactions: complex association and disassociation; irreversible: death and degradation). In most situations, reactions can be set to be irreversible during the first stage of the model development and

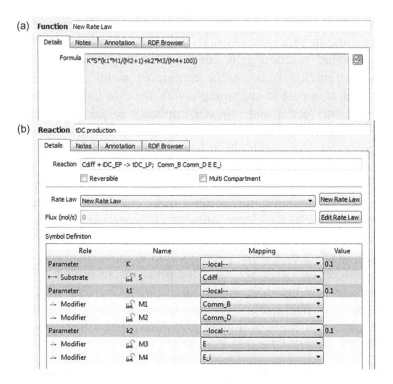

Figure 9.3 Reaction and rate laws in COPASI. The software allows the user to easily input custom rate laws to describe the included reactions. The variables are then mapped to model quantities and parameter values.

change during the model refinement process. In the *C. difficile* model, reversible reactions are used to incorporate plasticity between Treg and Th17 subsets (see Figure 9.3). As an exercise, you can attempt to assign a new rate law for the production of tolerogenic dendritic cells. Find the reaction iDC_E + Cdiff → tDC_LP. Click *"New Rate Law."* Enter the equation, $K*S*(k1*M1/M2 + k2*M3/(M4 + 100))$, into the "Formula" box and click the upper right button. Change the parameter descriptions so that K, k1, and k2 are parameters, M1, M2, M3, and M4 are modifiers, and S is substrate. Return to the reaction and select the rate law from the dropdown menu. Change the mapping so that Cdiff is S, M1 is Comm_B, M2 is Comm_D, M3 is E, and M4 is E_i.

Calibrating the model in COPASI: The most valuable data for the calibration and testing of a computational model is time course data. Additionally, almost all data must be preprocessed for the calibration purpose. For instance, on a cellular level, immunological data is often from flow cytometry; however, often the reported flow cytometry data

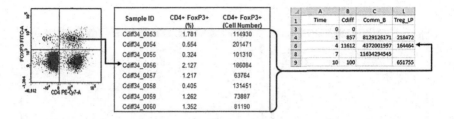

Figure 9.4 Sample calibration data pipeline. For models comprised cellular species, crucial experimental data is generated through flow cytometry. The output of many instruments will be percentage data. These data require conversion to cell number from the entire sample for the greatest utility in calibration. The data can be compiled into a single Excel file for import into COPASI.

is in the form of percentages and therefore must be converted to cell number whenever possible (see Figure 9.4). Furthermore, in the case of molecular level data, it is preferable to use protein-level data rather than expression-level data due to the nondirect relationship between transcript and molecular concentrations. Finally, data can be imported into COPSAI for calibration as average or data points; the program is customized to handle both types.

After compiling a sufficient amount of data, provide parameter estimates to get the model into a workable and functioning parameter space. Parameter estimated can be obtained from the literature, from newly designed experiments or from other similar models. Model calibration can then be used to predict more accurate parameter values. Although, it is also possible to manually enter and change parameters in COPASI, it would be more efficient if the process is systematized using time course simulation (under the tasks section in the left panel). Prior to running the simulation, click on *"Output Assistant"* (see Figure 9.5) in the bottom right and choose *"Concentrations, Volumes..."* under Plots and click *"Create."* This will allow you to create a graph of the simulation for all species. Click *"Run."* In the plot, click *"Hide All"* from the upper tool box, then specifically select the species of interest. It is generally recommended to start with one of the most upstream factors. Then, activate sliders, either from the *Tools menu* or the slider icon, which should be the fifth in the toolbar. Click *"New Sliders"* → *Reactions* → *Reaction Parameters* and select the reactions pertaining to your species of interest. Using the sliders, you can get the dynamics of the species close to the observations in the data. Finally, it is important to verify the steady state and ensure that model functions properly and does not exhibit nonsensical behavior.

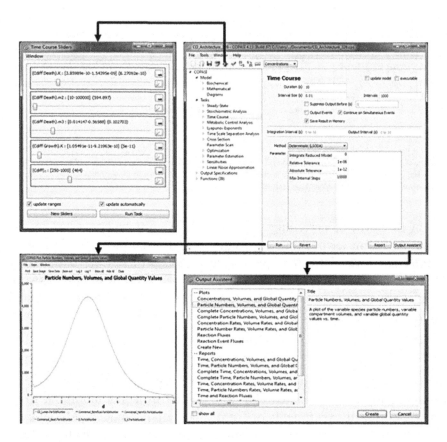

Figure 9.5 Preparation of the model prior to calibration. The time course and slider tools can be used to approximate the good initial guess required to accurately calibrate a model.

The model is now ready for calibration (see Figure 9.6). In the case of a large model, it may be best to break the model into sections rather than attempt to calibrate all parameters simultaneously. For instance, to calibrate the *C. difficile* model, we could start by calibrating the effector dendritic cells through Th17s and the tolerogenic dendritic cells through Tregs before calibrating them together and before calibrating them as part of the entire model. Also, it is possible to first save the previous set of parameters by clicking on the *Parameter Overview* option in the *Reactions* section of the left panel. In this window, you can click "*Save …*" in the lower right, which will save the entire parameter set within COPASI. The parameter set can then be accessed at a later time and reapplied to the model within the Parameter Sets option. The calibration process is carried out by

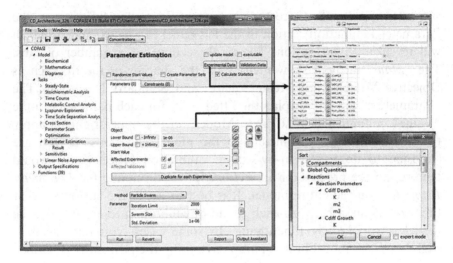

Figure 9.6 Parameter estimation process in COPASI. The task requires the input of experimental data and identification of parameters for which estimation is desired.

selecting "*Parameter Estimation*" from the *Tasks* section. You can compile your data in Excel with columns representing time and/or species (see Figure 9.4). The first row should contain species names. After saving the data as a tab-delimited text file, you can import the text file into COPASI by clicking the "*Experimental Data*" button. In the new window, click the button with the green plus associated with the "*File*" box and select your file. COPASI will automatically apply settings and select time course versus steady state based on the file uploaded. You will then need to select each column to be dependent, independent, or ignored data under type. Furthermore, it is important to match the model object with the column name. After completion, select "*Ok.*" You now need to select the parameters to be fitted and the admissible range for each parameter.

Select parameters by clicking the COPASI icon next to the "Object" box and choose the desired parameters from the pop-up. Because the model is refined with approximate parameters, the calibration process would fine-tune and optimize the fit; therefore, the upper and lower bounds should not be greater than two magnitude difference. After inputting the parameters and their ranges, select a *calibration algorithm* from the method dropdown menu. Certain algorithms may work better than others for a given model. For the *C. difficile* model, the Particle Swarm and Genetic Algorithm methods have shown to work well. Once the *Parameter Estimation* task is run, the Parameter Estimation section in the left panel can be expanded, which will reveal a *Result* option. The result section has a number of tabs. The *"Main"* tab will show metrics for the analysis of the fit, such as Objective Value, Root Mean Square, and Standard Deviation. The "Parameters" tab will display the fitted value for each parameter in the "Value" column. Click "Update Model" in the upper right to apply the new, estimated parameters to the model equations. If you are choosing to do a section-by-section calibration process, you would then repeat the process for all sections, prior to running the *Parameter Estimation* on the entire model. It is best to verify the steady state or time course tasks between each round of calibration to ensure that the model is still largely functioning. In some cases, you may need to slightly adjust noncalibrated parameters using the previously described slider method to repair the model if drastic changes occur.

Analyzing the model: Sensitivity analysis (SA) can be used for the analysis of the model. SA can highlight the most impactful parameters. SA can be performed prior to calibration to analyze only the network structure or following the calibration process in order to provide sensitivities focused on the calibrated parameter values. Local sensitivities can be performed within installed version of COPASI by using the *"Sensitivities"* task. To illustrate this process, we will run an analysis to show the effect of all local parameters on a given species during a time course (see Figure 9.7).

First, select *Time Series* as the subtask from the dropdown menu. Then, select *Single Object* as the effect. Next, follow the process, *COPASI logo button* → *Species* → *Transient Concentrations* → *[Cdiff](t)* → *OK*, to select your species of choice. Finally, set the *Cause* to be *Local Parameter Values* and click *Run*. Once the SA is complete, you will likely be automatically taken to the *Result* window; otherwise, you may expand the *Sensitivities* section and click *Result*. You can view your results in the window or export them using the *Save to File* button in the upper right. Most often, the scaled sensitivities are used for analysis purposes. Using the settings that were inputted, the higher the magnitude of the value, the more sensitive the species is to the parameter and the larger the impact alterations in the parameter will have. Positive sensitivities will indicate that an increase in the parameter value will increase the species concentration. Likewise, negative sensitivities will indicate that an increase in the

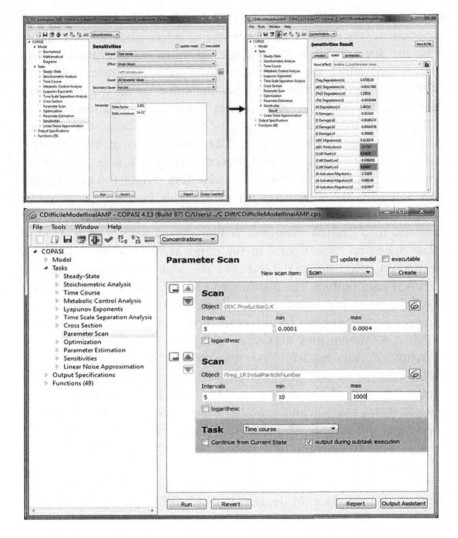

Figure 9.7 Model analysis. COPASI includes a number of tasks to aid in the analysis of the model including sensitivities and parameter scans.

parameter value will decrease the species concentration. Finally, global sensitivities can be submitted Condor-COPASI.

Performing in silico experimentation: Using a calibrated computation model, it is possible to design and perform an array of *in silico* experimentation to generate novel hypothesis. Not all findings during this process will be relevant or biologically feasible, but there are very few restrictions on the types of experiments that can be attempted.

One of the simplest experiments that can be explored is a knockout experiment. To execute this experiment, select your desired species from the Species section and change the initial concentration to zero. Ensure that either the values are saved as a parameter set within COPASI or that you can remember the values to return to the standard state. Within the selected species window, view the reactions that will produce the species. Then, go to each of these reactions and change parameter values to zero. These two steps will remove all of the species from the model and prevent their production. Then, run a time course to view the effects. A useful tool during the experimentation process is the *Parameter Scan* task. This task will allow you to quickly see the changes that occur in the dynamics of the model in response to a chosen quantity. Within the parameter scan window, select *Scan* and click *Create* in the upper right to apply a new scan item. Then, select the model quantity you wish to scan by clicking the COPASI logo button. The quantity can be an initial species concentration or a parameter value. Set the desired number of intervals, five is typically a good number to view a pattern. COPASI will automatically assign a minimum and maximum value to center around the value currently in the model. You may change the range if desired. Additionally, you may add multiple scans together, but ensure that the number of intervals for each scan is low so that the number of combinations is not overwhelming. Select *Time course* as the task and check the output during subtask execution. If it is difficult to see the results as they appear on your time course plot, export the data using the *Save Data* option on the toolbar of the plot. In the file, the data for the minimum value from start time to end time will appear on top. Beneath that set, data for the next interval will be present and so on.

In this exercise, the steps were presented in a linear manner but rarely will it proceed in as orderly in the development of new models. Very often, a good fit cannot be achieved through calibration, so the model equations need to be adjusted in an iterative process. SA can also be used to optimize the parameter range. Furthermore, it is important to compile more data for the calibration process whenever possible. Potentially, simulation results could create a desire to narrow or expand the focus of the network, and you cycle back to the first steps in the process. Finally, modeling is an iterative process and it will be important to be flexible and address issues that arise throughout the process.

Computational Model of the 3-Node T Helper Type 17 Model

Based on what has been explained so far in this chapter, the user should now be able to built a computational model and perform some of the tasks with COPASI. The second exercise is centered around the CD4+ T helper type 17 phenotype. The Th17 population is a key player in chronic inflammatory diseases such as inflammatory bowel disease, type 2 diabetes (T2D), rheumatoid arthritis, or in the infectious disease setting such as during *Helicobacter pylori* or *C. difficile* infection. Although Th17 cells have been highly characterized in the context of inflammatory pathologies, they remain elusive and controversial because of their plasticity, and many of their disease-causing mechanisms are not fully understood. However, it is widely accepted that Th17 cells are induced with a combination of IL-6 and TGFb, and that the main transcription factor during Th17 is RORgt. Indeed, the expression of RORgt leads to high production of IL-17A.

The computational model that will be created comprises the inductor of the phenotype (IL-6 and TGFb), the main transcription factor (RORgt), and the key cytokine produced by the Th17 cell (IL-17A). In the presence of the induction node, RORgt will be activated and IL-17A will be upregulated. The goal of the creation of this model is to represent these interactions between these Th17 players.

Creating models: Create a new model in COPASI using three species ("IL-6+TGFb", "RORgt", and "IL-17A") in one compartment. For this model, you can fix the inductor at a concentration of 1500 and RORgt and IL-17A will be set up as "reactions" with a concentration of 100. Ensure to select *"continue"* in order to create the different species (Figure 9.8).

Defining reactions: Create the two reactions: "Activation of RORgt" and "Production of IL-17A." The first one will involve the

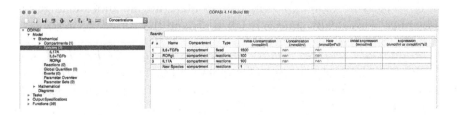

Figure 9.8 Model creation.

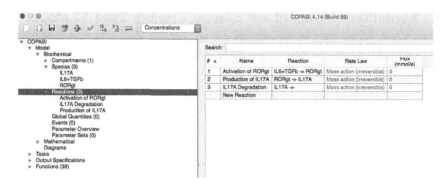

Figure 9.9 Defining the reactions.

inductor and RORgt, the correct nomenclature will be "IL-6+TGFb →
RORgt." This first reaction will be set up as a *Mass Action Irreversible*
with a parameter K = 0.1. The second reaction, which is the production
of IL-17A will allow RORgt to produce IL-17A. The exact nomenclature
will be "RORgt → IL-17A." This reaction will also be set up as a *Mass
Action Irreversible* with a K = 0.1.

Since the amount of IL-6 + TGFb is fixed, we can consider that
there will be a constant production of RORgt and therefore a constant
production of IL-17A. As a result, IL-17A will build up unless we set
up a third reaction that naturally degrades IL-17A. In COPASI, we set
up degradation reactions by leaving on one side of the equation empty.
The exact nomenclature will be "IL-17A →." We will set this reaction
again as an *irreversible Mass Action* with K = 0.1 as well (Figure 9.9).

At this point, the model would be set up and the user could start
performing different tasks, such as steady state analysis.

Steady state analysis: Click on *Steady State* and click *Run* with the
predetermined selections. You will observe that the system is able to
find a steady state where both RORgt and IL-17A are able to find a
state levelled at 1500 mmols/ml where there are no more changes in
dynamics. This steady state is reached around the 10-second mark.

Additional features and functionalities in COPASI: Using
COPASI, it is possible to select the output for displaying purposes. If
we click on *Output Assistant*, a list of different types of plots becomes
available to us. Let us click on Concentrations of all species and
quantities over time. In the menu options, click on *Time Course* and

perform a time course of 100 hours. In the resulting plot, we can observe the dynamics of IL-17A and RORgt over time. Please note that the induction node IL-6 + TGFb does not come up since we have it at a fixed concentration. Feel free to change it to reactions and play with the plot to observe a different dynamics on this node. *Sliders* are a good option to change the parameters in real-time. Click on the slider icon and select all the parameters of this computational model. If you play with the parameters, you will see how you are able to move the curves up and down.

Please note that both IL-17A and RORgt are able to reach steady state and stay at a specific concentration over time. The reason behind this sustained amount of these species goes back to the fact that the induction node, IL-6 + TGFb, is marked as fixed, therefore, unlimited. To see a different situation, go back to species and select *"reactions"* instead of *"fixed."* Go back to your *Time Course* and select a new plot in the *output assistant*. Next, run a *Time Course* and observe that a plot with the three species has been created. This time, however, you will observe that IL-6 + TGFb is now part of the plot and that the species do not conserve that high and steady level over time. In contrast, now these species are being upregulated and then degraded over time, shaping the dynamics of these reactions as bell curves.

The last task to be highlighted is the *Parameter Scan*. The scan changes the concentration of different molecules that you can specify over time in a continuous manner. Please click on the Scan and then select *Time Course* in the dropdown menu. We will change the concentration of the inductors IL-6 + TGFb with a range 1−1000. Click on *Output assistant* and select the scan plot and click create. You will see how the plot is now created in real-time. The scans will allow you to determine how an increase in concentration changes over time. For example, in this case, you can see how the more inductor, the more RORgt and the more IL-17A. This is an obvious result, but it allows us to learn how to run scans. Scans can reveal interesting behaviors in more complex computational models. In the scan plot, we will find the increasing concentrations in the x-axis and the concentrations of the nodes of interest in y-axis. If we take a closer look at the scan plot, we can observe how the inductors IL-6 + TGFb form a direct correlation. This is because we are scanning these two nodes. In the case of RORgt and IL-17A, we can observe how more the IL-6 + TGFb, the more RORgt and IL-17A concentrations.

Computational Model of the 9-Node Th1/Th17/Treg Model

This next exercise will show you how to create a 9-node model that is also related to CD4+ T-cell differentiation. The model we will create will contain three different CD4+ T-cell phenotypes: Th17, Treg, and Th1. These three phenotypes will be differently characterized by the way we will induce them, the transcription factors that will get activated, and finally the cytokines or other soluble factors that the phenotypes will produce. At this point, you are familiar with the Th17 induction: IL-6+TGFb together will induce expression of RORgt, and such expression will drive IL-17A production. In the case of Th1, the inductor will be IL-12. IL-12 will activate a transcription factor named T-bet. T-bet is the trademark of the Th1 phenotype, and it is widely accepted that high expression of T-bet leads to high production of interferon gamma. We will also represent that last part in our model. Last, the regulatory phenotype Treg will be induced with TGFb, and the transcription factor that will drive the final production of IL-10 will be FOXP3. You can see the network created using CellDesigner in Figure 9.10. Also remember to include a degradation reaction for the

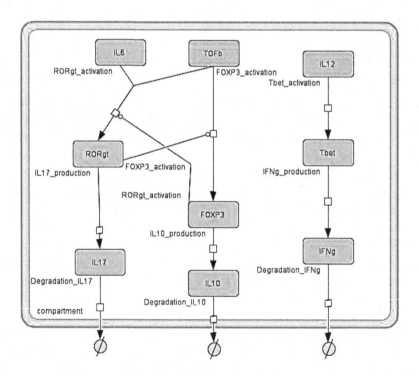

Figure 9.10 The 9-node model of the CD4+ T-cell differentiation.

three final products: IL-17A, IFNg, and IL-10. Please note that there is a common inductor between Th17 and Treg, which is TGFb. Look at the figure to see how you can separate IL-6 and TGFb and have different systems of induction. In contrast to Th17 and Treg, Th1 will be an independent factor in this system. Finally, some of these phenotypes will be interconnected. Note how RORgt and FOXP3 are also connected through an inhibition reaction. Please set up an inhibition from FOXP3 to the activation of RORgt, and from RORgt to the activation of FOXP3. Remember that to set up inhibitions, you go from a node to a reaction.

In order to implement this model into COPASI, open a new file and start adding species. We will add first the three inductors: IL-6, TGFb, and IL-12. These three inductors should be created with a fixed concentration of 100 mol/l. Second, create the transcription factors with an initial concentration of 1 mol/l and marked as "reactions," since we will create the reactions that will upregulate the transcription factors. Finally, let us create the cytokines: IL-17, IL-10, and IFNg. Very similar to the transcription factors, the cytokines will be created with an initial concentration of 1 mol/l and marked as "reactions."

Next, let us create the reactions that will drive the concentrations of these factors up and down. In this case, we will follow *Mass Action* for all the reactions except for the activation of FOXP3 and RORgt. In this case, we will use the *Hill Function*. The Hill function has demonstrated to work very well in reactions involving different inhibitors. In our case, the activation of FOXP3 is inhibited by RORgt, and the activation of RORgt is inhibited by FOXP3. In order to set up the Hill Function, the first step is to create a *Global Quantity* named *Hill* with a value of 2 (see Figure 9.11). This will be our Hill factor in the equation.

Next, we will take a look at the reactions to see how we can set them up. For convenience, we can set all of them up as *Mass Action* for now and then create the *Hill function* in the next step. Figure 9.12 shows the details in all the reactions created.

If we double-click on top of FOXP3 activation, we will see the details of this reaction. In *Rate Law*, you should see how *Mass Action (irreversible)* has been selected. Click on *"New Rate Law."* We will manually enter the *Hill Function*. This reaction has one substrate

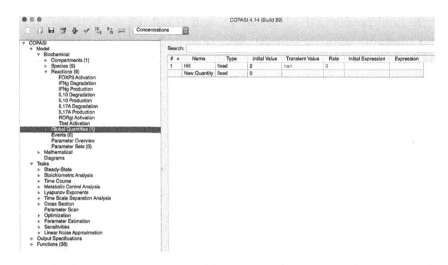

Figure 9.11 Defining reactions using global quantity.

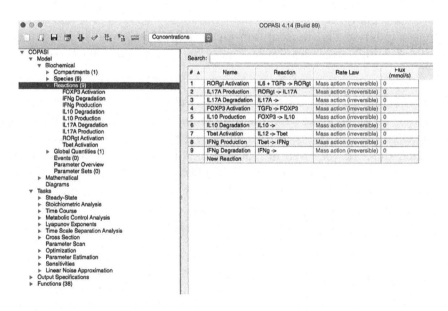

Figure 9.12 Reaction equations for the 9-node Th1/Th17/Treg model.

(TGFb), one product (FOXP3), and one modifier (RORgt, which inhibits the reaction). Take a look at Figure 9.13 to see how to set up the formula.

If you click Commit, it should look like Figure 9.14.

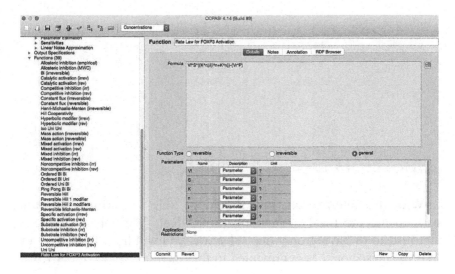

Figure 9.13 Setting formulas in COPASI.

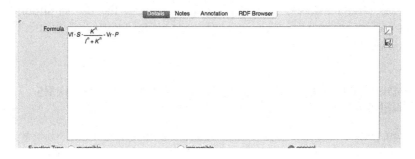

Figure 9.14 Formulas in COPASI.

You will see that under *Parameters*, you can select the *function* or *description* of each one. All of them need to be marked as Parameters except for *S* (marked as Substrate), *P* (mark as product), and *I* (Inhibitor, mark as modifier). Click *Commit* and go back to the reaction with FOXP3. Now you will be able to select *Rate Law* for FOXP3 Activation under the dropdown *Rate Law Menu*. You will see that COPASI populates the different parameters. The only change you need to make is map "*N*" to *Hill*. For that, click on the dropdown menu for "*N*" in the mapping column and select the *Global Quantity* that you created before: "*Hill*." This will allow you to control the Hill coefficient to any number you want by just changing your Hill parameter.

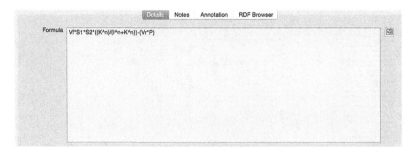

Figure 9.15 Formulas in COPASI.

With this information, you should be able to perform the same steps to prepare the Hill function for RORgt. The only difference is that instead of having only one substrate, you will have two (IL-6 and TGFb). This should be represented in the function (see Figure 9.15).

With all these settings on place, you should be able to start giving different initial concentrations and perform *steady state analyses, time-courses,* and *sensitivity analyses.* We recommend the use of sliders, so you can observe how changing different concentration can affect the outcome of the system.

MODEL COMPLEXITY AND MODEL-DRIVEN HYPOTHESIS GENERATION

When generating a new model, an important question is what would be the optimal size and complexity? As with a large number of modeling decisions, the answer depends heavily on the question the model is being designed to answer. In cases when a single informative parameter or equation is the desired end result or if an in-depth mathematical analysis is thought to be required, a small model of 10 species or interactions would likely be best suited for the purpose. However, when predictive capabilities and insights into novel interactions are important, a more expansive model will provide the best results. Nonetheless, the initial choices in model building do not need to create inflexible limits on the size of the model throughout its lifespan. A model can expand and contract to fulfill a variety of functionalities. For instance, the development and analysis of a cytokine-driven signaling network has been informative about the roles of numerous molecules on and the general status of CD4+ T-cell differentiation and plasticity. However, to analyze the development and maintenance of a

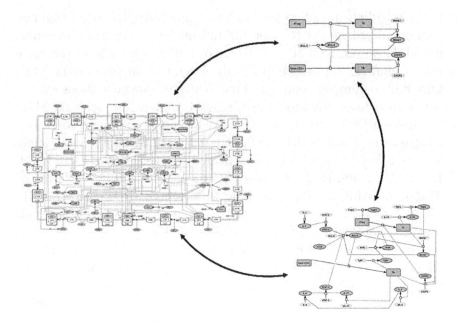

Figure 9.16 Cyclical progression between models of different sizes.

specific population of T-follicular helper (Tfh) cells, the full model may not have been the most ideal. Tfh cells can differentiate similar to other CD4+ T-cell subsets, but the expression of a receptor upon differentiation targets the Tfh population to a specific location. In this location, the effects of the systemic environment are partially lessened. Therefore, the local environment is predicted to have a larger effect on the ability of this population to persist. Additionally, the ability of this population to switch from low levels to chronically elevated levels suggests that a bistable nature could be central to the interaction network driving the production of the Tfh population. Combined, these two factors suggested that a small network may be most suitable for initial investigations. Furthermore, once the initial analysis was complete, the model was re-expanded to an intermediate state to restore the potential of novel contributor and interaction discovery (Figure 9.16).

One of the main strengths of smaller models is its ability to handle the equations analytically without the need for an ODE solver or similar software. To display this, simply attempt to assemble an equation for Bcl-6 activation from the networks. On the surface, there is very little difference in complexity between the three models. At first glance, the intermediate model appears to be the most complex with five modifiers compared to the two for the full model and one for the small model. However, next attempt to remove other species from the equation so that Bcl-6 production is only dependent on parameters rather than both parameters and variables. While all three equations expand within their respective models, the massively interacting scale on which the full model is constructed is unwieldy and prohibitive to further analysis. In the full model, the Bcl-6 is activated by STAT-3 and inhibited by Blimp1, but STAT-3 is activated by IL-6, IL-9, IL-10, IL-21, IL-22, IL-23, and IL-27. Picking just one of these, IL-22 is affected by TGFβ and AhR. Continuing, AhR is influenced by IL-2, TNFα, IL-27, and so on. Even on the small scale, the one equation with one modifier would expand to include parameters connected to every species in the model: Bcl-6 to Blimp1, Blimp1 to Tfr, Tfr to nTreg and CXCR5, CXCR5 to Tfh, and Tfh to naive CD4+. When dynamics with nonlinearities are placed onto a network such as this, even the small model is reaching the limits of what can be comfortably handled without specialized software such as COPASI or Matlab.

Attempts to reduce model equations creates a cascade of substitutions. The need for further model simplifications raises doubts over the perceived usefulness of small models for mathematical analysis (see Figure 9.17).

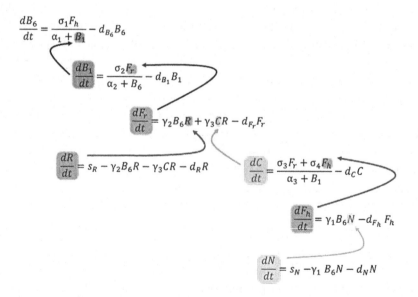

Figure 9.17 Equation complexity of an interconnected network.

A crucial first step to condensing a larger model into a smaller model or to expanding in the opposite direction is modifying the architecture of the model. Through knowledge of your network or a literature search, you will be able to identify the most important elements of a larger model that should be retained through the reduction. For example, in the development of Tfh cells, the transcriptional regulators Bcl-6 and Blimp1 have key antagonistic roles, so any model describing the differentiation and stability of the Tfh population should find a way to incorporate these molecules. An additional consideration with this model during the simplification was the ability of the model to possess bistability. For bistability or behaviors such as oscillations, feedback must be present within the network. Therefore, the mutual inhibition between Bcl-6 and Blimp1 had a second layer of importance added. But with the removal of many of the cytokines and signal transducers during the reduction, many of the elements necessary to determine a phenotype of the cell were also removed. Consequently, the network was modified to compensate by explicitly creating species that could show occurrence of differentiation.

Alternatively, a way to generally reduce a larger model is through SA. By analyzing the sensitivity of the desired quantity (i.e., activation of Bcl-6 in the Tfh model) to all parameters, it is possible to identify the least impactful parameters and simplify the reactions to which they belong. For example, the production of IL-10 from Tfr cells activates the production of TGFb, which in turn forms a complex with its receptor (TGFbRC). The complex then activates the RXR species. However, after an SA on the network, the parameters associated with the production of IL-10 and TGFb are determined to have sensitivities approximately 100-fold greater than those associated with complex formation. This result is a good indication that the complex formation step could be merged with the production of TGFb with little impact on the rest of the network (see Figure 9.18).

The sensitivity of TGFbRC formation is significantly lower than the sensitivity of IL-10 and TGFb production; therefore, the formation of TGFbRC step was merged with the preceding step.

In contrast, there are two primary ways of expanding a model beyond the simple addition of one or two reactions: you can add around the existing model that will allow you to retain the core behavior and parameters exhibited by the smaller model or you can expand reactions

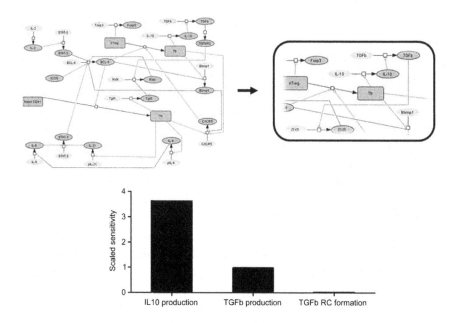

Figure 9.18 Model reduction through sensitivity analysis.

to include intermediate processes that might have been ignored in the initial model which could create a more biologically descriptive model. When adding to a smaller core model, it is relatively simple to observe the effects that additions will have on the network behavior. However, during the expansion process, each step could alter the overall behavior of the system, and this alteration can be undesirable. If the original model contains behavior that is satisfactory and accurate, it is best to attempt to retain similar feedback loops through the expansion process. The process of calibration can also inform if a model could benefit from further expansion; for instance, if the calibration data set may be sufficient and contain valid data but a good fit cannot be obtained. Additionally, if the time course simulation for a species does not closely resemble the observed experimental data or a steady state for the system might not be reachable, then the model might need further enhancements. This could indicate that a change in the model dynamics is necessary either through manipulation of the ODEs in the system or through the addition of a new species or interaction.

Finally, a small model can seem easier to solve analytically (and sometimes that is true); however, the predictive power of larger calibrated models are unquestionably more relevant in a clinical setting.

Larger models can also be used for more complex *in silico* experimentation and hypothesis generation. Smaller models on the other hand can provide new insights into basic science research and represent the building blocks for larger and more comprehensive models. Finally, dynamics of larger models can also provide valuable information on the temporal behavior of various components and could be used to build predictive models for treatment regime and have valuable clinical and pharmacological relevance.

CONCLUDING REMARKS

Modeling highly complex systems that are well calibrated with experimental data can be valuable and drive experimentation towards unforeseen and nonintuitive directions. However, building computational models that are comprehensive and calibrating these models with different data types can be a daunting task without using the proper tools and techniques. This chapter provides a set of hands-on examples that are at the cutting edge of the immunoinformatics practices with tools that are highly specialized and freely available. The ultimate goal of the modeling processes presented is to empower wet-lab researchers to perform modeling and revolutionize the way wet-lab immunology research and discovery are performed.

ACKNOWLEDGMENT

This work was supported in part by National Institute of Allergy and Infectious Diseases Contract No. HHSN272201000056C to J. Bassaganya-Riera and funds from the Nutritional Immunology and Molecular Medicine Laboratory (www.nimml.org).

REFERENCES

[1] Hoops S, et al. COPASI—a COmplex PAthway SImulator. Bioinformatics 2006;22 (24):3067—74.

[2] Meier-Schellersheim M. SIMMUNE, a tool for simulating and analyzing immune system behavior. Hamburg: University of Hamburg; 1999.

[3] Folcik VA, An GC, Orosz CG. The Basic Immune Simulator: an agent-based model to study the interactions between innate and adaptive immunity. Theor Biol Med Model 2007;4:39.

[4] Mei Y., et al., ENISI MSM: a novel multi-scale modeling platform for computational immunology. In: 2014 IEEE International Conference on Bioinformatics and Biomedicine; 2014. pp. 391—396.

[5] Mei Y.G., et al., ENISI SDE: a novel web-based stochastic modeling tool for computational biology. In: 2013 IEEE International Conference on Bioinformatics and Biomedicine (BIBM); 2013.

[6] Mei Y., et al., ENISI Visual, an agent-based simulator for modeling gut immunity. In: IEEE International Conference of Bioinformatics and Biomedicine (BIBM); 2012.

[7] Sklar E. NetLogo, a multi-agent simulation environment. Artif Life 2007;13(3):303—11.

[8] Tisue S., Wilensky U. Netlogo: a simple environment for modeling complexity. In: International Conference on Complex Systems; 2004. pp. 16—21.

[9] Collier N, Howe TR, North MJ. Onward and upward: the transition to Repast 2.0. In: Proceedings of the first annual North American association for computational social and organizational science conference 2003. Pittsburgh: Carnegie Mellon University.

[10] Funahashi A, et al. CellDesigner 3.5: A versatile modeling tool for biochemical networks. Proc IEEE 2008;96(8):1254—65.

Printed in the United States
By Bookmasters